NATURAL REMEDIES FOR SLEEP

NATURAL REMEDIES FOR SLEEP

ESSENTIAL OILS, MEDITATION, ACUPRESSURE, AND MORE FOR A GOOD NIGHT'S REST

Dr. Kye Peven, ND, DSOM

Illustrations by Christy Ni

ROCKRIDGE
PRESS

For general information on our other products and services or to obtain technical support, please contact our Customer Care Department within the United States at (866) 744-2665, or outside the United States at (510) 253-0500.

Rockridge Press publishes its books in a variety of electronic and print formats. Some content that appears in print may not be available in electronic books, and vice versa.

Interior and Cover Designer: Liz Cosgrove
Art Producer: Samantha Ulban
Editor: John Makowski
Production Editor: Rachel Taenzler

Illustrations © 2021 Christy Ni

ISBN: Paperback 978-1-64739-647-3 | eBook 978-1-64739-648-0

R0

CONTENTS

INTRODUCTION

We spend, on average, one-third of our lives sleeping.
And yet, for some of us, sleep can feel difficult, elusive, or down-
right impossible. When was the last time you got in bed before
midnight, fell asleep easily, slept through the whole night without waking up, and awoke feeling rested and refreshed in the
morning? Perhaps you can remember a time when sleep was
like this. Or maybe this experience of sleep is something you've
never had, and you can only imagine what it would be like.
Maybe you sleep well, but you have a partner, family member,
or friend who has difficulty sleeping. No matter what your relationship is to sleep, this book will provide helpful advice and
information on natural ways to improve your sleep.

I was initially drawn to health and medicine through
a desire to understand my own life experiences. Though I
thought I might work as an engineer, a series of experiences
with meditation early in life showed me that happiness is
much more closely connected to health than to material
possessions or technology. I found myself more and more
wanting to understand how *people* worked, instead of how
things worked. Conventional medicine, with its narrower focus
on disease and dysfunction, wasn't able to satisfy my desire
for a medical system that integrated every level of human

experience, from physical to spiritual. However, I didn't want to abandon the incredible detail and analytic capacity of Western science. Naturopathic medicine was the perfect combination, and when integrated with a classical understanding of Chinese medicine, provides me with an extremely comprehensive understanding of human health.

This book begins with a general overview of sleep: what it is, why it's necessary, what types of benefits come from good sleep, and what can go wrong when sleep issues occur. Next, we will look at the concept of natural remedies and gain insight into what makes them distinct from more conventional types of sleep remedies, such as medications. Once we have created some context, we will then get you set up with a sleep toolkit. The toolkit chapter (page 26) reviews the specific resources you will need to start getting a good night's sleep, and how to prepare for this daily journey into the land of slumber.

The next several chapters will discuss specific remedies. For each chapter, you will learn how and why the remedies work; for each individual intervention, we will discuss the rationale behind the remedy, take a brief look at some of the scientific evidence, and see how it may work for you. Of course, not every remedy is appropriate for every person, which is why we will cover a great many potential remedies that you can use. Finally, in the last chapter (page 140), we will discuss specific sleep situations you may have experienced or are experiencing, as examples of how to apply the remedies in the previous chapters.

Though I am sure the material in this book will be of value to you, it is not a substitute for professional medical advice. Don't be afraid or embarrassed to reach out for additional help, or to get confirmation about the usefulness of a particular therapy for yourself.

HOW TO USE THIS BOOK

This book is meant to be used as a reference. Each technique or remedy presented includes clear indications of when to use it, instructions for how to use it, and potential cautions. You do not have to read through the entire book before checking out a particular therapy. However, gaining a deeper understanding of sleep will only be to your benefit. In particular, some of the lifestyle modifications discussed in chapter 2 (page 14) are the most valuable elements in ensuring a good night's sleep. Without setting yourself up for a good night's sleep, many of the more specific therapies will be less effective. If you don't intend to read through this book in its entirety, I urge you to go through chapter 2 at a minimum.

I hope this book proves valuable and useful to you, and that after reading it you have the resources you need to start getting the excellent sleep you're seeking.

CHAPTER 1

AN INTRODUCTION TO SLEEP

Welcome to the first step on your path to good sleep! In this chapter, we will cover the basics: what is sleep, why do we need it, and what happens when we don't sleep well. We will also define what makes a remedy or therapy *natural* in order to compare natural remedies to more conventional treatments, such as medications. Near the end of this chapter, you will find a basic self-check for your current quality of sleep, which will be a valuable metric as you begin implementing some of the remedies in later chapters. By returning to this self-check, you will be able to see how your sleep has improved.

WHAT IS SLEEP?

We have all experienced sleep, and most of us have observed other people or animals sleeping, so we all have a basic idea of what sleep feels and looks like. *Sleep* can be defined as "the natural, easily reversible periodic state of many living things that is marked by the absence of wakefulness and by the loss of consciousness of one's surroundings."

In humans, the muscles relax during sleep, so we tend to sleep lying down with our eyes closed. Sleep is also characterized by changes in our brains. Our brains produce electromagnetic waves, and for alert, waking consciousness, these waves are around 12 to 40 Hz (waves per second) and are known as beta waves. Waves from 8 to 12 Hz, known as alpha waves, occur during REM (rapid eye movement) sleep and are associated with dreaming. Theta waves, from 4 to 8 Hz, and delta waves, below 4 Hz, happen during deep sleep.

Our Circadian Rhythm

Circadian rhythms refer to ways in which life keeps time over a 24-hour period. Our circadian rhythm helps regulate our sleep-wake cycle, stimulated primarily by ambient light and melatonin. Melatonin, a hormone secreted by the pineal gland, is produced in both the brain and the gut; in the brain, it is one of the signals that increases sleepiness. During the day, exposure to light suppresses melatonin production. As evening approaches, the light from the sun starts to dim, and this signals the pineal gland to start producing melatonin.

In addition to suppressing the production of melatonin, bright, full spectrum light also helps regulate sleep in other beneficial ways. However, this presents certain challenges in our technologically advanced society, since most of us are surrounded by sources of artificial light, especially at night. Historically, humans weren't exposed to light much stronger than a few candles at night. The relatively recent (and drastic) change in our evening light exposure may be influencing our ability to sleep well.

THE BENEFITS OF A GOOD NIGHT'S SLEEP

The most important benefit of getting adequate, good-quality sleep is feeling good! But sleep also has numerous other benefits, both short-term and long-term.

Short-Term Benefits

On a daily basis, getting enough quality sleep keeps the mind and body functioning well. While we're sleeping, the energy spent on being awake and aware is redirected to crucial metabolic functions, helping us heal from the wear and tear of daily life. This allows the body to clean up metabolic waste products, rebuild damaged cells and tissues, regulate our hormone levels, manage our immune systems, and much more.

Similarly, all of these functions are happening in the mind. During sleep, the various thoughts, emotions, and experiences from the day are sorted, categorized, and integrated into long-term memory. This is another way of saying that sleep is necessary to transform what has happened *to* you into *who* you are. Good sleep also contributes to mental clarity, concentration, and increased creativity; the common term "sleep on it" refers to the ability of the mind to come up with new perspectives, ideas, and solutions to previously unsolvable problems.

Long-Term Benefits

Sleep is one of the cornerstones of good health. Health, in its broadest conception, is much more than the absence of disease. Good health is the ability to flexibly adapt to life, at the physical, emotional, and mental levels. It means having the energy and ability to do what you want to do, whether that is reading a newspaper or climbing a mountain. And good health makes you less susceptible to disease, both acute and chronic.

In Chinese medicine, sleep is required to restore yang energy. Yang is required for all activity, as it represents the basic ability of an organism to *act*, to make something happen. As a person ages, they are able to generate less and less yang energy. In general, children are much more energetic than the elderly. Children also need more sleep, and this allows them to be as energetic as they are while awake. Sleep creates the possibility of action, of energetic functioning, and ultimately the possibility of life.

WHY AREN'T WE SLEEPING?

There are a myriad of reasons why we might find it difficult to sleep well. One big reason has to do with the sensitivity of our circadian rhythm to light, as mentioned earlier (page 2). We live in an ocean of artificial light, coming from both indoors and outdoors, as well as from multiple screens. Also, by working inside, we miss the opportunity for bright, natural light exposure during the day.

Another reason has to do with stress. We live in a world now where the pace of life has increased dramatically, and where we often find ourselves constantly attempting to complete a to-do list that never ends. Along with money stress, relationship stress, and more, this contributes to difficulty relaxing enough to fall, and stay, asleep.

Other reasons for sleep issues include the noise that permeates our cities, work schedules such as shift work, unhelpful eating habits, substance use, medication side effects, and much more.

COMMON SLEEP STRUGGLES

The following are some of the more common reasons people have trouble sleeping.

Anxiety and the Future

Do you lie awake at night worrying about the future? Perhaps it is all the things you need to do in the coming days. Or it's anxiety about bad things that could happen, or what might be coming in the near future. This anxiety often happens before a momentous event, such as a performance or presentation, or before traveling. It prevents people from falling asleep, and can also trigger waking up in the middle of the night. The mind races, and sleep doesn't come.

Rumination and the Past

Some people have trouble sleeping because their minds are busy thinking of the past. It's common to ruminate on things you could have done or said differently. Perhaps it's difficult for you to fully "digest" the experiences from the day, and therefore it takes time to process them mentally before you're able to fall asleep. Or you're filled with regret at what could have been. Either way, the mind continues to "chew" on these thoughts, and sleep is difficult.

Restlessness and Agitation

Sometimes people are physically restless. This can accompany mental restlessness, but can also occur purely at a physical level. Restless leg syndrome is one conventionally recognized disorder that can affect sleep. People can't seem to get comfortable, feel restless and fidgety, or toss and turn all night. This makes deep sleep hard to achieve.

Hypervigilance

Hypervigilance stems from past trauma, which we have all experienced to some degree or another. Trauma, defined simply as an experience that was perceived as life-threatening, can create a state in the body where the perception of danger is constant. The mildest form of this is when someone is a light sleeper, and wakes with the slightest sound. The more severe forms make it difficult to sleep at all. When it feels like there is potential danger at every moment, losing awareness of one's surroundings in order to fall asleep becomes a bad idea.

Chronic Pain

Of course, some people have trouble sleeping simply due to the fact that some part of their body hurts most or all the time. Chronic pain is often due to multiple causes, such as prior injuries, overall cardiovascular fatigue, and overwork. Since sleep is necessary to heal and rejuvenate the body, when chronic pain prevents good sleep it can create a vicious cycle, where lack of sleep contributes to the ongoing pain.

Heartburn

Many people experience acid reflux, or heartburn, when they try to lie down and go to sleep. This is often associated with eating late in the evening, or eating while stressed, which weakens digestion. The burning pain in the stomach, chest, or throat can be very uncomfortable.

WHEN TO SEE A MEDICAL PROFESSIONAL

If after you've tried many of the therapies and remedies in this book and nothing seems to have changed, consider seeking professional help. If you suspect your sleep problems are due to an underlying condition, such as chronic pain, headaches, acid reflux disease, or a mental health issue, see a medical professional. It is also advisable to see a professional if you are taking sleep medications, or if you are taking other types of psychiatric medications such as antidepressants, antipsychotics, antiepileptics, or anxiolytics.

Dealing with trauma is often easier with assistance. If you know you have trauma in your past, finding a trauma-informed practitioner might be the best action you can take for yourself.

THE CHALLENGES OF POOR SLEEP

Earlier in the chapter, we looked at the benefits of adequate sleep. Now let's take a look at what happens when we don't get enough sleep.

Short-Term Effects

Acute sleep deprivation, such as staying up all night, is associated with numerous negative effects on both the mind and the body. At the mental level, lack of sleep leads to negative changes in mood, attention, short-term memory, and other cognitive abilities; it can also increase anxiety, depression, and the formation of false memories. Physically, it can lead to decreased motor control and reaction times, making us clumsy, and making it more dangerous for us to drive or operate machinery. Of course, not sleeping enough can lead to falling asleep during the day. Car crashes due to drivers falling asleep are common.

As sleep deprivation increases, people start to experience psychotic symptoms, such as altered perception, anxiety, irritability, and changes to their sense of time—all the way to hallucinations and delusions. These typically go away once the person sleeps, but for some people, these symptoms may persist.

Long-Term Effects

Chronic lack of sleep has now been documented to influence the development of many health conditions. Sleep debt over time activates our stress-response system, resulting in issues similar to what happens with chronic stress. Due to the negative effects on the immune system, this leads to more infections and more inflammation, which increases the risk of many common conditions, such as diabetes, heart disease, and cancer. At the mental level, chronic lack of sleep can both cause and worsen anxiety, depression, bipolar disorder, ADHD, and other mental health issues.

NATURAL REMEDIES 101

A *natural* remedy can be thought of as anything that comes directly from the natural world and exists on its own without having to be synthesized by humans. Natural remedies can include plants and plant extracts, minerals, and substances present in the body (like melatonin), as well as physical and mental exercises. Another way to conceptualize a natural remedy is to consider if the remedy would exist without any advanced technology. If it could have existed hundreds of years ago, it's probably natural.

NATURAL REMEDIES VERSUS PHARMACEUTICALS: PROS AND CONS

Natural remedies and pharmaceuticals each have their advantages and disadvantages, which depend on how they're commonly used and how their effects are understood.

Pharmaceuticals are almost always single chemicals that are meant to either change, overcome, or replace normal body function. They work through force and have to be taken in sufficient quantity to make things happen in the body. There is little consideration given to what the body does as an adaptation to the presence of the drug. This pharmaceutical action is both an advantage and a weakness. These powerful substances can suppress symptoms, often almost immediately, but only while they're in the body. As soon as you stop taking the drug, symptoms often return, and sometimes stronger than before, as the body reflexively pushes back against the action of the drug.

In contrast, natural remedies such as herbal medicines are often not taken in high enough quantities to act in a drug-like fashion. They are typically not as strong as pharmaceuticals, either. Instead of changing or suppressing symptoms through force, a natural remedy causes the body to change as it responds to the remedy's presence. At times, this response can be immediate, but often it takes longer to experience results.

However, because this is the body's adaptive response, it persists even after the remedy is no longer present.

One other major distinction is that pharmaceuticals, even when used correctly, often cause side effects, which are the body's response to the strong *push* given by the drug. Natural remedies, because they focus on the *response*, often have fewer side effects. When someone has side effects to a natural remedy, it is often a sign that the remedy is being used like a drug, or the remedy is not right for that person.

THERE IS NO MAGIC BULLET

Sleep is a skill, and like all skills it cannot be instantly mastered but gets better with practice. As a natural process inherent to the complex phenomenon that is life, sleep is not a switch that can be turned on and off, but rather an intricate process with many different causes, influences, and obstructions. There is no single therapy or magic substance that can instantly grant perfect sleep; any claim to the contrary should be examined very carefully.

GREAT SLEEP IS WITHIN YOUR POWER

Great sleep may be effortless once mastered, but building the necessary muscles of sleep takes work. This is work I hope you're gladly willing to undertake, as good sleep is a natural birthright of all human beings. No matter how difficult sleep currently is for you, no matter how long it's been since you experienced a good night's sleep, know that rejuvenation and vitality are available, and likely closer than you think.

BASIC SELF-CHECK: HOW IS YOUR SLEEP?

- I typically go to sleep before midnight and sleep for seven to nine hours.
- When I get in bed, it takes me less than 15 minutes to fall asleep.
- Once I fall asleep, I stay asleep the whole night.
- I wake feeling rested and refreshed.

If you disagree with any of these statements, your sleep could likely be improved.

CONCLUSION

Though we may feel quality sleep is beyond our grasp, the knowledge and work required to achieve good sleep is not. Though the work may be unfamiliar and difficult at times, the reward is more than worth it. The rest of this book will give you the knowledge and tools you need to start on your journey to feeling better, more vital, and healthier than you can imagine.

CHAPTER 2

SET YOURSELF UP FOR A GOOD NIGHT'S SLEEP

Certain environments and activities are conducive for sleep, whereas others disturb sleep. This chapter will go over the basics of how to create an environment that will make sleeping easier and more restful. Implementing these suggestions will make the remedies in the subsequent chapters much more effective. If changing your lifestyle to incorporate everything in this chapter is too much to do all at once, start with one or two sections. Then try to pick another section to work on every week. Soon you'll find you've been able to make a significant and positive change in the quality of your sleep.

SUNSHINE

As discussed in the previous chapter, exposure to bright, full spectrum light during the day is very helpful for restful sleep. Light during the day helps maintain our circadian rhythm and prepares us for sleep when it gets dark. It's important to obtain this light from natural sources; even on a cloudy day the intensity of outdoor light is often many times greater than the light in a standard indoor workplace. If you cannot spend some time outside during the day, try at a minimum to find an indoor space at home or at your workplace with large windows that let in a significant amount of light. Get as much bright light during the day as you can.

LIGHTING AT NIGHT

Just as it's important to get bright light exposure during the day, it's also important to reduce bright light exposure at night. Without a reduction in light intensity, the body doesn't understand that it will soon be time for sleep. Ideally this means that at least two to three hours before bedtime, the brightness of artificial light is reduced in order to mimic the darkening of the skies as the sun sets.

Another factor is the color of light we are exposed to in the evening. It's known that blue light suppresses melatonin production more than yellow, orange, or red light. Blue light exposure in the evenings is thus more detrimental to sleep than warmer colors. To help set the stage for good sleep, it's important to reduce blue light exposure after dark, such as from screens and fluorescent or LED lights. When using mobile devices and screens at night, use night shift mode or apps to filter out blue light.

For best sleep, the bedroom should be as dark as possible. Any electronics that emit light should be turned away from the bed, turned off, or removed from the room. Keep night-lights as dim as possible and place them where the light is not visible from the bed. Use thick curtains (or blackout curtains) to prevent streetlights from shining in through any windows.

HYDRATION

Hydration is important at all times, including overnight and during sleep. The effects of dehydration are well known, and include symptoms such as dry mouth and throat, fatigue, brain fog, headache, anxiety or irritability, dizziness, muscle cramps, and more. The body loses a significant amount of water overnight, which cannot be replaced during sleep. Furthermore, dehydration is correlated with reduced sleep time; studies have shown people who sleep only six hours on a regular basis lose more water than people who regularly sleep eight hours. Dehydration is also correlated with sleep apnea, since a person loses more fluids when breathing through the mouth compared with breathing through the nose.

It's important to go to sleep properly hydrated. However, drinking too much right before bed can lead to having to get up in the middle of the night to go to the bathroom. Therefore, it's best to try and stay hydrated throughout the day. If you forget to drink during the day, try and hydrate in the early evening, so you don't find yourself dehydrated when you're about to go to sleep.

MEALS AND EATING

The digestive system has a major influence over sleep. We now know that the gut contains a second "brain" (often referred to as the enteric nervous system), a neural network that is in constant communication with the brain in our head. The gut produces the majority of our neurotransmitters (chemical messengers in the nervous system), typically many times more than compared with the brain. If, when, and what we eat in the evening and before bed all play an important role in sleep.

In general, going to bed on a full stomach will make sleep more difficult. One common issue is mechanical: if you tend toward heartburn or acid reflux, lying down on a full stomach will often make this worse. However, even without any reflux, attempting to sleep and digest at the same time doesn't usually work so well. This is because sleep is a time of rest and rejuvenation, whereas digestion is an activity (even though it's happening inside the body). The body is busy digesting, which doesn't leave enough energy or attention to perform all the necessary sleep functions. As a rule, you should stop eating at least two to three hours before going to sleep. If you get heartburn at night, stop eating at least four hours before sleeping.

There are, however, some people who sleep better if they eat right before bed. These are people who tend to have trouble keeping their blood sugar up. If you are the kind of person who needs to eat every few hours; if you get irritable, dizzy, faint, or weak when you get hungry; or if you find that you otherwise suffer if you go too long without eating, you will do better with a snack before going to sleep. Eat a small but filling amount of food (no junk food or sugar) before you go to sleep. A small amount is what fits in the palm of one hand.

Vitamins and Minerals

It is beyond the scope of this book to discuss sleep-nutrient interactions in detail, but know that many nutrients are involved in sleep, and deficiencies (or excesses) in any of them have the potential to create issues. Nutrients known to have an impact on sleep include vitamins A, B_6, B_{12}, C, D, and E; iron; zinc; copper; potassium; magnesium; and calcium. Interactions among nutrients are also important, such as the synergy between all the fat-soluble vitamins (A, D, E, K) and balance between various minerals (for example, taking too much calcium can create magnesium deficiency).

The best way to achieve balanced nutrition is to eat a nutrient-dense, plant-based, diverse, whole foods diet. Reduce or avoid processed foods, junk food, refined cooking oils, and chemicals in food as much as possible. For recommendations on supplementing your diet with individual nutrients, it's best to see a professional.

READING

Many people read in the evening as a way to wind down and relax before sleep. This is a great strategy, but there is a caveat. It is important not to read in bed if you have trouble falling or staying asleep. You want to associate the bed with sleeping, so if you like to read in the evening, do it somewhere other than the bed. Then, when you get sleepy, put the reading material down and get into bed. Remember, all the rules about lighting still apply, so make sure you're using a warmer, dimmer light source for your reading.

COMFORT AND COLORS

Sleep is a state of relaxation, so it's important that the bedroom feels comfortable and cozy. According to feng shui principles, the bed should be positioned so the doorway is not in line with the bed, especially with the head of the bed. Also, covering up at night is very important, even if it's only a light sheet. The covering provides a sense of protection for the body while consciousness is turned inward, and keeps the minute changes in your physical environment from disturbing you. The color of the bedroom is also important, though some people are more sensitive to color than others. The best colors for sleep are neutral to warm, from off-white to earth tones to shades of orange, yellow, or red. It's best to avoid cooler colors such as blues or purples unless you have a strong personal preference, as these tend to stimulate mental activity.

TEMPERATURE FOR SLEEP

It's well known that our core body temperature fluctuates throughout the day and that falling asleep is accompanied by a drop in body temperature. This drop is facilitated by keeping the bedroom cool so that the body isn't overheated when it's time for bed. Sleeping in a hot environment, especially if there is also high humidity, decreases sleep quality and time spent in deep sleep.

According to a review of sleep habits in the *Presse Medicale*, the optimal bedroom temperature is about 60 to 65 degrees Fahrenheit. Warmer than 75 degrees or colder than 55 degrees and sleep will not be as good. However, individuals are different, and the best temperature for you may not be within the 60- to 65-degree range. Experiment so you know what works best for you.

Warming Yourself

Even though our core body temperature drops as we fall asleep, our skin temperature rises as blood flows to the peripheral tissues. As the body relaxes in preparation for sleep, the hands and feet will warm up. If your hands and feet are cold, this process will take longer, and it will also take longer to fall asleep.

Warming the feet and keeping them warm at night increases sleep quality. Taking a hot foot bath before sleep can be very helpful, especially if your feet are often cold when you go to bed or you find yourself wearing socks to sleep. Warming the feet relaxes the nervous system and assists the body in changing the temperature dynamic from the daytime state. Fill a bucket, tub, or even a large pot with hot water, and place your feet in for 5 to 10 minutes, or until they feel very warm. This is best done immediately before sleep, so you can get right in bed afterward. (A more advanced version of this simple therapy, titled Warming Socks, is detailed on page 93.)

THINGS TO AVOID FOR A BETTER NIGHT'S SLEEP

Now that we've discussed some good practices for sleep preparation, let's review some things that are better to avoid.

Caffeine

For most people, consuming caffeine later in the day will make it hard to fall asleep. There are those who can drink coffee in the afternoon or evening and still sleep just fine, but for the majority of us it is best to avoid caffeinated beverages in the second half of the day. If you are especially sensitive to caffeine or other stimulants, you may need to limit all caffeine consumption to before noon.

Alcohol

Despite its popularity as a way to relax, alcohol is actually very disruptive to sleep patterns. Drinking alcohol in the evening may help you fall asleep more quickly and has been shown to increase slow-wave sleep, but after the effects wear off sleep becomes disturbed in the second half of the night. This rebound effect is more pronounced the more drinks you have;

the strongest evidence of sleep disruption is with binge drinking and those with alcohol dependency. You will sleep better if you are no longer under the influence of alcohol by the time you go to bed, which means drinking less and drinking earlier in the evening.

Sugar

Refined sugar is best thought of as either a medicine or drug, or perhaps a seasoning agent, rather than food. When we consume more than a teaspoon of sugar, the body has to quickly secrete insulin to prevent blood sugar from rising too high. This rapid response can create an overcorrection, causing blood sugar to drop too low, which triggers the secretion of cortisol and adrenaline to rebalance sugar levels. Cortisol and adrenaline are both secreted in times of stress and danger and are stimulating, and they will keep you awake. Furthermore, sleep requires a stable blood sugar level, and this back and forth from high to low is detrimental to solid sleep.

Naps Late in the Day

Naps can be a wonderful way to recharge and rejuvenate during the day, but sleeping too long later in the day can interfere with nighttime sleep. The best time for a nap is in the early afternoon, and naps should not be longer than an hour. If you have a dip in energy later in the afternoon, resist the urge to take a long nap, and limit your nap to 10 to 20 minutes.

Exercise at Night

Exercise late in the day can interfere with sleep in several ways. Because exercise requires activity, it directly counters the need to wind down in the evening. Exercise also raises our core temperature, which is the opposite of what happens as we move toward sleep and rest. For these reasons, it's best not to exercise within three to four hours of bedtime.

WHAT WORKS BEST FOR YOU?

As you go through this book, take note of remedies and therapies that draw you in, and ones that you feel resistance toward. Go over the recommendations in this chapter, and pick one or two to work on to start. Try a therapy or two from later chapters that are easy and doable. Don't force yourself to implement something unpleasant or uncomfortable. Find out which approaches work best for you.

SHIFT WORK

Because of the close connection between light and wakefulness, shift work can be very stressful to our system. Managing your light exposure is the most important element of creating a healthy sleep schedule when you have to work at night. It is imperative to create total darkness in your sleeping space, so daylight does not disturb your sleep. It's also best if you can get bright, full spectrum light when you first wake up in the afternoon or evening and reduce bright light in the morning before you go to sleep. This will help mimic the natural light-dark cycle.

CONCLUSION

The elements discussed in this chapter are the foundation of good sleep. The remedies and therapies presented in chapters 4 to 9 will be especially useful if they are based on this foundation. In the next chapter, we will gather a toolkit of sleep aids that will help prepare you to implement the more specific therapies that follow.

CHAPTER 3

YOUR SLEEP TOOLKIT

Before you choose and use individual therapies, it will be helpful for you to have a general overview of the types of tools and equipment you may need. Think of this chapter as a master list for the actual materials you'll need in order to implement many of the specific therapies in the chapters that follow. Since you may be unfamiliar with some of these tools, we will also discuss where to find them, and, if necessary, how to distinguish good quality from poor quality.

As you go through this chapter, keep in mind that you don't need everything mentioned here. After you've read through the later chapters to discover which remedies and therapies are appealing to you, come back to this chapter to find out where and how to acquire any materials you may need.

ITEMS YOU'LL FIND HELPFUL TO GET STARTED

Some of the following items will need to be purchased, but many of the tools to facilitate better sleep are things you likely already possess. Others you may be able to find for free, or for very cheap, at second-hand or thrift stores.

Sleep Tracker

The technology to track sleep has progressed enormously. Sleep studies that used to require extended stays in facilities with specialized equipment have given way to wristbands and smartphone apps. There are numerous ways to track sleep, from filling out a spreadsheet to wearing a headband that monitors your brain waves. If tracking is important to you, there are a few things to consider.

The gold standard for sleep tracking is direct measurement of brain waves. There are now several commercially available devices that can do this. These will give you the most accurate sleep data, but they are quite expensive. The next most accurate items are a variety of wearable and nonwearable devices that track heart rate, breath rate, body movement, sound, and other factors, in order to estimate how much and what type of sleep you are getting. They typically require a connected smartphone to interpret the data generated from the device; they are moderately priced, though not cheap. There are also apps that you can use with a smartphone that don't require an external device, and simply use the phone's capacity to detect sound and movement to monitor your sleep. Finally, tracking your sleep can be as simple as filling out a spreadsheet.

MANUAL SLEEP TRACKING

If you intend to track your sleep manually, you'll want to capture at least the following data points:

- The time you get in bed
- About how long it takes to fall asleep
- How many times you wake up
- If you wake for a particular reason:
  - Bathroom
  - Emotions
  - Dreams
- How long it takes to fall back asleep (and if it takes a long time, what stops you from falling back asleep)
- What time you wake in the morning
- If you feel rested after sleep

Try to record this data first thing in the morning, when you wake up, before you forget.

For any sleep tracker you decide to purchase, make sure to get a device you'll actually use. If you spend hundreds of dollars for a headband that monitors brain waves, but you don't like sleeping with something on your head, the device won't do you any good. Remember to read reviews, because some devices don't work as well if you sleep with a partner. Take the time to find a device that will work for you.

Mattress, Sheets, and Blankets

It may be obvious, but important physical elements for good sleep include the mattress, sheets, and blankets or comforters. If you're physically uncomfortable in bed, then it will be harder to sleep well. Pay attention to the material of your bedding, and if you are sensitive to chemicals you may want to invest in organic sheets. If you sleep better with a heavy blanket, you may find weighted blankets helpful. If you tend to overheat at night, you'll most likely need a different setup than if you get cold easily.

Herbal Teas

Though commercially available herbal teas at most grocery stores are convenient, most brands are relatively low quality, containing low-grade herbal powder that oxidizes and goes stale quickly. It will be worth your while to investigate any local herb shops in your area; many natural food grocers also carry bulk herbs. If there is nothing in your area, look for a reputable online merchant that carries high-quality, chemical-free herbs.

Essential Oils

Essential oils (EOs) can be found at many natural food grocery stores, herb shops, and natural pharmacies. They can also be found easily online. Because essential oils are so concentrated, it is especially important to ascertain whether the oils are made from plants grown without pesticides, herbicides, or other chemicals. Also, make sure the oils do not contain synthetic fragrance and that any carrier oils used are of high quality. You don't want to be breathing in these chemicals, as many of them can be quite toxic. Before you buy anything, spend a few minutes learning about essential oil testing and quality control, and contact the essential oil company you want to purchase from to ask them how they verify essential oil identity and quality.

Candles

The warm and low intensity light given off by candles is an excellent way to wind down at night. You may find scented candles that you enjoy, or you may prefer unscented candles, such as simple tealights. If you choose to use candles, you should also have a fire extinguisher on hand in case of an emergency. Also, place candles where you will not bump into them or knock them over, and be aware of any drapes or other hanging materials that could catch fire. Never place a candle underneath anything flammable, and never leave a candle unattended.

White Noise Machines and Music

Many people who are sensitive to disturbances and wake easily find that soft white noise can be very helpful. There are multiple white noise machines on the market, and if you find that noises often wake you at night, a white noise generator may be a useful tool (apps can also fulfill this function). Music can help you wind down and relax in the evening, and if you find it helps you fall asleep, then playing this music at bedtime can be a good idea. A bedtime playlist can become a helpful part of your routine, and after a while you will start associating this music with getting a good night's sleep. Once this happens, you will be able to use this playlist to make yourself sleepier in anticipation for bed.

A Journal

Keeping a journal is very useful. The journal can be as simple or as elaborate as you desire, from a plain spiral-bound notebook to a handmade journal with personal illustrations on the cover. The act of writing engages more of the brain associated with memory formation than typing on a screen or keyboard. Though you may be tempted to make notes on a mobile device or computer, a physical journal is superior and recommended.

Humidifier

If you live in a dry climate, or your bedroom is dry due to either indoor heating or cooling, a humidifier could make your sleep much more comfortable. Reasons to run a humidifier include waking up feeling dry or dehydrated, waking with a sore throat, knowing you tend to snore, or knowing you often breathe through your mouth at night. Make sure to clean the humidifier regularly to prevent algae or mold growth.

Fans

In hot climates, sleeping with a fan on is very common, especially if air conditioning is unavailable, or if you dislike the feeling of air conditioning. If you have a fan in the bedroom, it is best to set it up so it doesn't blow directly on you while you are in bed, as this can lead to summer fevers and sickness. Set up the fan to circulate the air in the room indirectly.

Soundproofing

If you are especially sensitive to noise, or you live close to regular noise (such as a train route), you may find that an extra effort toward soundproofing your bedroom will be well rewarded. This can range from hanging some fabrics to absorb sound all the way to rebuilding the walls with insulating materials. What will be necessary and effective will depend on the sources of noise, your current sleeping space, and how sensitive you are.

CONCLUSION

Now that you have a basic toolkit, it's time to get into specifics. The following chapters will introduce many different techniques, activities, therapies, and remedies. As you read about them, consider that combining techniques from different categories will be more helpful than implementing several from the same category. Find the ones that appeal to you and give them a try. You will be on your way to better sleep!

CHAPTER 4

CBT STRATEGIES FOR UNDERLYING ISSUES

Cognitive behavioral therapy (CBT) refers to using the mind consciously to change a behavior, emotion, or thought. Though it wasn't always a specific therapy the way we think of it, learning to be aware of our thoughts and consciously changing our patterns and habits has been a staple of religious and spiritual traditions for millennia. Recommendations in the previous chapters could be considered CBT strategies, such as dimming lights in the evening. In this chapter, we'll examine more specific things you can do, both before you get in bed and when you are already in bed and are having difficulty falling asleep.

A BRIEF HISTORY OF CBT

CBT arose in the mid–20th century as a reaction to behavioral therapy, the predominant type of therapy at the time (which focused only on behavior and did not include thoughts). It wasn't initially called "CBT," but the basic premise was the same: instead of responding directly to an event or situation, we respond to the thoughts and emotions the event generates. By changing our perspective, we can thereby create a different internal response.

WHEN IS CBT USED?

CBT can be used for all kinds of things, as the core element is the link between perception, belief, and behavior. The latter are present in most of our daily activities, and thus the techniques introduced in this chapter can actually be applied beyond sleep. CBT is useful for changing unhelpful responses to stress and for developing new habits and patterns of behavior that serve your happiness. CBT can also be used to help establish better eating habits, exercise routines, reducing or quitting use of various substances, and more.

THE BENEFITS OF USING CBT

CBT has been shown in many studies to be very helpful for changing behavior, including unconscious behaviors like sleep (Mitchell et al. 2012). Though CBT can be hard work, you already have everything you need inside yourself; there's no need for additional tools or expensive devices. All you need is a willingness to change something about yourself. Once you learn new habits (of both thought and physical behavior), these new and more useful patterns will usually sustain themselves, as they become part of your everyday life. So even though it can be difficult at first, once you've successfully implemented a CBT technique, it tends to become easier and easier to maintain.

HOW CBT CAN HELP YOU SLEEP BETTER

Just like almost everything else in your life, sleeping is a skill, and CBT can train you to sleep better. There are so many obstacles in our modern lives to getting quality sleep, ranging from the presence of artificial light everywhere to anxious thoughts that keep us up at night. CBT can help you successfully navigate these obstacles. Although remedies such as essential oils address the body's physiology and unconscious mind, CBT is about using your conscious mind to influence itself and your body's physical state. Our minds are powerful, and learning to use the mind effectively can help bring about positive change.

HOW TO USE CBT FOR SLEEP

We have actually already discussed a few CBT techniques, such as dimming the lights before bed and regulating the temperature in the bedroom. These are both ways of exerting conscious control to change the environment around you. CBT for sleep centers around associating certain triggers with sleep and removing signals for wakefulness. In this way, you train your subconscious mind to associate the right place, time, and mental state with good sleep.

STRATEGIES

Don't try to practice all the following techniques at once. Pick a few to implement, and once they become second nature, you can try adding more. Start with the easiest ones, as completing them will create a feeling of success, which will make the harder ones easier to tackle.

SCHEDULING CONSISTENT SLEEP

Our modern disconnect from the rhythms of nature contributes to the difficulty in establishing regular sleep. It is therefore important to have a regular sleep schedule in order to regulate our body's response in the face of artificial lighting and our sometimes 24-hour activity.

If at all possible, it is best to go to sleep and wake up at the same time every day.

It is essential to associate bedtime with sleepiness, which is an important reason not to take late afternoon naps. Initially, creating a schedule may be difficult, but it's generally best to set a firm wake-up time as the first step. It is almost always easier to wake up at a new time than to force yourself to fall asleep at a time you're not accustomed to. As your system gets used to waking up at a certain time, you will start feeling tired when it's time to go to sleep in the evening. Initially, make sure to wait until you're ready for sleep before getting into bed. This may mean getting less sleep until your body adjusts, but it will help you associate bedtime with sleep, as you don't want to get in bed knowing that you're going to lie there awake.

If your wake-up time is 7:00 a.m., don't allow yourself to fall asleep at 8:00 p.m., either. This is important if you tend to fall asleep early in the evening, only to sleep poorly or find yourself awake in the middle of the night. Going to bed too early has the same effect as taking a late nap, so resist going to bed until seven to nine hours before your wake-up time.

HOW MUCH SLEEP DO I NEED?

People need different amounts of sleep, but most adults need between seven and nine hours. Remember the self-check in chapter 1 (page 13). If you're sleeping only five hours, but you fall asleep easily, sleep through the night, and wake feeling rested and refreshed, that's probably enough.

Note: Falling asleep easily means without sleep aids, and rested and refreshed in the morning means *without* coffee or other stimulants.

LIMITING SCREEN EXPOSURE

Two big factors that interfere with sleep are light and activity. Unfortunately, mobile devices, televisions, laptops, and screens in general are sources of both. The light and movement coming from screens is quite stimulating; with our increase in screen time, this presents a significant obstacle to getting good sleep.

It's best to be screen-free for at least 30 minutes before bed, and preferably 60 minutes or even longer. If you lose track of time in the evenings, setting an alarm can be a good way to regulate screen time. There are also apps that can help you monitor your device usage. Instead of watching videos, listen to a podcast or audiobook so you aren't looking at a screen before bed.

If at all possible, keep screens out of the room where you sleep. If this is not possible, keep screens out of the bed itself—don't be on your device browsing social media or watching online videos. Also, don't watch television while in bed. If you are looking at a screen in the evening, make sure to turn down the brightness, and use a blue light filter. Falling asleep in front of a screen is not a good sleep option; the light coming from the screen will interfere with your body's ability to fully relax into deep sleep, and your sleep quality will suffer.

GETTING UP IF YOU ARE AWAKE

It's generally better to keep all activities out of the bed, except sleeping and sex. You want to associate your bed with sleeping, and if you are doing other things in bed, there's a danger that the bed will become associated with these activities instead. If you are in bed and can't fall asleep, don't stay in bed for more than 20 minutes. Get up and do something else. Many of the techniques in this book can be done at these times. Remember to avoid bright or blue light so you don't promote wakeful-ness and disturb your circadian rhythm. When you feel ready to fall asleep, then get back into bed.

PLANNING FOR TOMORROW

Many people find they have trouble falling asleep because their minds are full of things that need to get done. Planning in your mind for the next day or for the future can create anxiety that prevents sleep, or it can simply occupy the mind enough that falling asleep doesn't happen. A busy mind can occur when you're ini-tially falling asleep and if/when you wake in the middle of the night.

If this is your experience, one excellent strategy is to keep your journal handy so you can create to-do lists. By writing down the things that need to get done, your mind will be relieved of the need to remember every-thing, which should make it easier for you to relax and fall asleep. Be as detailed with your notes as you need to be to satisfy the part of your brain that is preoc-cupied. If you wake up and realize you've forgotten something, just write it down and go back to sleep.

Upon reading through your to-do list in the morning, you may find that you don't actually have to accomplish everything on the list. You may also find that the list is helpful in structuring your day. If you don't use the list that day and the important activities from the night before haven't stayed in your mind, recognize that the worry over your tasks may not be about the tasks themselves, but about something else. Figuring out what the root cause is will go a long way toward helping you calm your mind when it's time to sleep.

ACTIVATING HEART COHERENCE

In cultures all around the world, the heart is considered the center of our emotional experiences, especially emotions related to our connections and relationships with others. The emerging research around heart-rate variability and coherence is beginning to validate this perspective (McCraty 2015). *Heart rate variability* (HRV) refers to how our heart rate changes over time and is a sensitive measure of coherence; *coherence* refers to the state when the heart, mind, and emotions are all integrated and in alignment.

Increasing heart coherence has multiple benefits, but one of them is increased emotional stability, otherwise known as calm. Since falling asleep typically requires this sense of stability, increasing your heart

coherence before bed can be very helpful for a good
night's rest.

CONNECTING TO THE HEART

- Place your attention on the area of your heart (the
  center of your chest).

- Take a breath into this area, extending the breath
  slightly to a count of five to six seconds in, and then
  five to six seconds out.

- As you continue to breathe into this area, begin
  activating a positive feeling, such as a sense of appre-
  ciation, or a sense of care for yourself or others.

- Focus on the physical and emotional feeling of
  this positive energy as it manifests in the area of
  your heart.

- Repeat for 5 to 10 breaths, or for several minutes.

AFFIRMATIONS

Affirmations are a way to replace negative or unhelpful
thoughts with positive ones. Using affirmations involves
saying, either out loud or silently in your head, a phrase
that expresses a belief you want to have about yourself.
Affirmations are especially helpful if your inner dialogue
is based in language, as opposed to imagery or more
abstract concepts.

WORDS OF AFFIRMATION

- I am loved

- I am blessed

- I am provided for

- I am enough

- I am worthy

- I am beautiful

- I am complete

Choose a phrase from the previous list, or make up one of your own. Use your existing thoughts as a guide to chart the direction you want to take your mind. If you have habitual thoughts around how much you have to do, you could use a phrase such as "I am at rest" or "I am fulfilled." Repeat your affirmation phrase for one to five minutes.

RELEASING REGRETS

It's common to lie awake at night thinking over past regrets. Whether they are recent or distant, all regrets involve interpreting a past experience as "bad," thereby passing judgment on yourself. It is important that we learn from our mistakes, but self-castigation is never helpful. If you find your mind stuck in the past, the following process can help you restructure your thoughts. An example of this process can be found on page 46.

- Ask why. Pretend a good friend is with you asking you why you feel regretful. Your friend doesn't understand your feeling in the slightest, so you have to explain it. Explain why your regret is *bad*.

- Take your answer and ask why again. Keep asking why until your answer is something that can't be explained, that just *is*.

- Ask yourself: this thing or state that just *is*, is it really true? How do I know it's true?

- If this thing or state is not true, then what could be true instead? Come up with one or more believable statements as alternatives to this thing that *is*.

- If these alternatives are true, how does that change your perception of the event or experience that precipitated the feeling of regret?

**A COMMON REGRET IS NOT GETTING
ENOUGH DONE**

1. I feel regret because I should have been
   more productive.
2. I should be more productive because otherwise I'm
   lazy. (This could be the defining statement, or you
   could continue with further why's.)

   a. Being lazy is bad because it means I'm a
      bad person; I'm a bad person when I don't
      work hard. OR
   b. Being lazy is bad because I need to keep
      up with my coworkers; I want them to think
      highly of me. OR
   c. Being lazy is bad because I'm in danger;
      working hard is the way I keep myself safe from
      other people.
3. Is it true that people think I'm lazy?
4. What else could be true?

   a. People don't have any opinion of me at all, since
      they're busy with their own lives.
   b. I'm actually very productive according to others.
   c. Working hard doesn't really make me feel safer;
      maybe the danger is due to something else.
5. Maybe I'm reading too much into things and I don't
   need to feel bad about my day.

If you have little regrets from the day, you may be able to go through this process quickly, or even skip the initial steps and simply hypothesize about different interpretations of the events of the day. If you have large regrets, this may be an ongoing process, in which case you'll want to make use of some of the other techniques in this book to help you fall asleep.

BEING KIND TO YOURSELF

When we lie awake at night with thoughts swirling through our heads, how often are they thoughts of love, compassion, and kindness? Being kind to ourselves is powerful when we've been taught to be cruel or judgmental.

Being kind to yourself means accepting who you are, with all the imperfections and flaws that you come with. It means not judging yourself when you're anxious, when you can't fall asleep, or when you're lying in bed reading your phone knowing that you're not supposed to. It means remembering that you are human, and you are doing the best you can.

Think of yourself as a small child. It is usually acceptable for children to make mistakes or feel intense emotion, because this is how they learn. When a child is having a difficult time, kindness helps more than yelling or criticizing. At the same time, one doesn't let a child "get away" with bad behavior. Similarly with yourself, you can be both kind and strict, if necessary.

If you notice patterns in your thoughts or behavior that are making it hard to sleep, from anxious thoughts to late-night screen time, begin the process of changing these patterns—but be kind to yourself as well. You can even hang a sign reminding yourself to practice kindness. Recognize that the way you feel and the things you do were for a good reason initially. They just don't serve you anymore, and so you'll make changes, at the pace that works for you.

GENERATING GRATITUDE

Gratitude and kindness go hand in hand. Gratitude can arise spontaneously, such as when receiving a gift, but can also be increased through regular practice. Gratitude expands the heart field and naturally counteracts stress, negativity, anxiety, and depression. Research has shown that gratitude can increase a sense of well-being and happiness, as well as contribute to better sleep. By increasing your capacity to experience gratitude, you can generate a sense of calm that will help when it is time to go to sleep.

Generating a sense of gratitude effectively requires a connection to the heart. HeartMath, an organization studying the physical, mental, and emotional impact of the heart, has shown that it is the heart that creates this field of positive energy, and thus connecting the mind to the heart is very helpful (McCraty 2015). For best results, establish heart coherence first before continuing with this exercise (see "Activating Heart Coherence," page 42).

Whether you have done the heart coherence exercise or not, generating gratitude is remarkably simple.

MATERIALS
A journal or notebook
A pen or pencil

INSTRUCTIONS
1. Every night before going to sleep, write down three to five things you are grateful for in your journal or notebook.
2. If you cannot think of three to five things, write at least one.
3. *Optional:* Spend one to three minutes focusing on the feeling of gratitude while connected to your heart.

4. If after this exercise you have trouble falling asleep, continue to focus on the feeling of gratitude while lying quietly in bed.

PROGRESSIVE MUSCLE RELAXATION

Physical tension in the body often reflects mental and emotional stress, and if the body is tense it will be more difficult to relax enough to fall asleep. Progressive muscle relaxation takes you through the body, part by part, helping you direct your conscious will toward letting go of tension at a physical level. This exercise is best done when you are already lying down in bed.

INSTRUCTIONS

1. Begin by placing your attention on your feet. Notice if you are holding tension in your ankles, feet, or toes. Since you are lying down, there is no need to engage any of these muscles. Allow yourself to release any tension or tightness you notice.

2. Move to the calves and lower legs. Notice again if you are subconsciously tensing any muscles in this area, and if so, release it.

3. Continue in this way, moving from the calves to the thighs and hamstrings.

4. Next, focus on the buttocks and area of the pelvis.

5. Move to the lower back, then the mid-back.

6. Notice any tension in the abdomen. Are you holding in your belly? If so, let it go.

7. Bring your awareness to the chest.

8. Move to the upper back and shoulders.

9. Allow your awareness to move down the arms, ending at the hands and fingers.

10. Come back up to the neck and throat.

11. Finish with the face and head.

As you move through the body, if you have a hard time drawing your attention to a part of your body, use the illustration on pages 52–53 as a guide. If you notice tension but find yourself unable to release it, contract the muscles in the area as hard as you can for five seconds. Then release, and notice the sensation of relaxation. If you still notice tension, then just keep your awareness on that area for a short time, and allow the tension to remain without fighting against it. You cannot force tension to release, so if your body isn't ready, just allow it to remain for now.

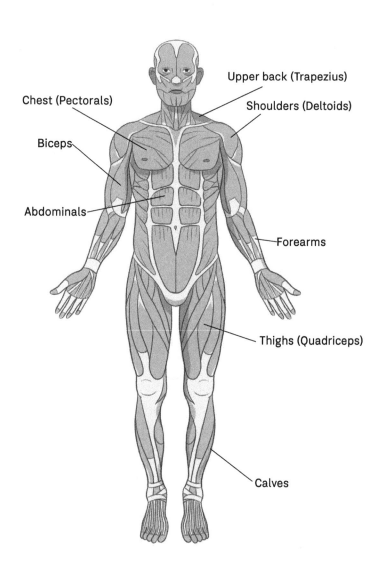

Upper back (Trapezius)

Chest (Pectorals)

Shoulders (Deltoids)

Biceps

Abdominals

Forearms

Thighs (Quadriceps)

Calves

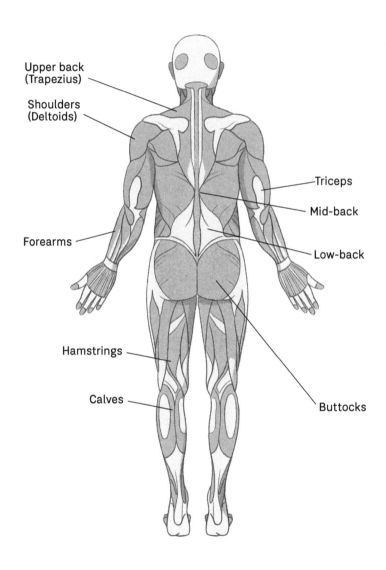

Upper back
(Trapezius)

Shoulders
(Deltoids)

Triceps

Mid-back

Forearms

Low-back

Hamstrings

Calves

Buttocks

CONCLUSION

All the techniques presented in this chapter will help you prepare for a good night's sleep. They will also help you establish a
solid foundation for good health overall. If you find that none of
these exercises appeals to you, or you've tried them and don't
seem to find much benefit, don't worry, as the following chapters will present many more exercises and remedies. The next
chapter will focus on meditative techniques and will introduce
exercises that make use of the mind to help create good sleep.

CHAPTER 5

MEDITATION, MANTRAS, AND VISUALIZATIONS

Meditation is a time-honored technique for exploring and experimenting with consciousness. Though there is significant overlap between cognitive behavioral therapy (CBT) and meditation, CBT is more focused on changing thought patterns and habits of behavior, whereas meditation tends to focus on self-awareness and shifting the nature of the mind itself. Because meditation is about self-inquiry, the experience of meditating is necessarily unique to each individual. This chapter will help you find a way of meditating that suits you well.

THE POWER OF YOUR MIND

Western science is beginning to recognize what philosophers in the Eastern world have always known: the mind is of utmost importance in our health and is as strong (or stronger) an influence as anything we do at the material level. In Chinese medicine, the highest level of doctor treats the *shen*, the human spirit consciousness. Decades of research at the Princeton Engineering Anomalies Research (PEAR) lab has shown that human intention has small but measurable effects on machinery. Even though we've all been taught that what happens only in our minds can't have an impact on the outside world, this is not true.

The mind has an even greater impact on our internal world. By exerting the power of our consciousness, we can do wondrous or terrible things to ourselves. The placebo effect, long thought of as a nuisance (because it interferes with objective findings), is actually an incredibly powerful tool for healing and transformation. One study showed that even when participants were told they were taking a placebo, the act of taking a pill every day had over 50 percent of the effect of taking the actual medication, when compared with no treatment at all. Our minds are so much more powerful than we've been led to believe.

THE BENEFITS OF MEDITATION, MANTRAS, AND VISUALIZATION

Given that the mind is our most powerful tool, wouldn't you like to understand it better, strengthen its power and ability, and make use of it appropriately? Just as physical exercise strengthens the body and is important for physical health, mental exercise strengthens the mind and improves our mental health. The techniques introduced in this chapter will help you develop a degree of mastery of your mind, helping you strengthen this often-neglected aspect of yourself.

These mental techniques have also been used for millennia for the work of enlightenment and spiritual development, such as becoming closer to God or merging with cosmic unity. The use of meditative techniques for that purpose is beyond the scope of this book. However, even though they've been used for spiritual purposes, these techniques will still be very helpful for the more mundane goal of getting a good night's sleep.

HOW TO USE MEDITATION FOR SLEEP

The mind is heavily involved in the process of sleep, and interventions that target the mind (which is different from the brain) can have a significant influence. For many of us, it is the mind that prevents us from falling asleep; using meditative techniques to calm the mind and direct our consciousness into the body are very helpful.

Even if you don't fall asleep immediately by using these techniques, they will still be helpful. Sleep is a time of rest and recovery, and by keeping yourself in a meditative state, you can achieve similar benefits, even if you don't completely fall asleep. However, do not try to substitute meditation for sleep. Some of these techniques are best used before bed, whereas others can be done when you are already in bed, and occasionally in lieu of sleep, if done correctly.

TECHNIQUES

As you read through the following techniques, pay close attention to what the technique is attempting to accomplish, as they do not all have the same goal. You may find yourself gravitating toward a particular technique, whereas others seem difficult or useless. Start with what works for you.

In addition, many techniques will be helpful for creating mental calm and increased focus throughout the day, and are not only meant to be done right before bed. If events and stress during the day have less impact, you won't have to work as hard at night to wind down. Consider spending some time practicing these techniques in the morning in order to help you sleep more soundly in the evening.

APP-GUIDED MEDITATIONS

There are countless meditation apps available, and new ones come and go. If you're just starting to explore meditation techniques, having someone guide you through the experience can be very helpful. With so many different apps to choose from, you may want to keep the following in mind:

- Some apps contain different types of meditations for different purposes: calming anxiety, relaxation, gratitude, and so on. Be sure when you select an app that it has the types of meditations you are seeking.

- Apps can feature bells, gongs, and even nature sounds. If simple and rhythmic sounds are soothing to you, an app of this kind may be a good choice.

- Meditations for sharpening focus and concentration will be more helpful in the morning, whereas meditations for calming anxiety and increasing relaxation will be more helpful in the evening. Of course, if you are often stressed in the morning, the more calming meditations may be just as helpful to use in the morning as in the evening.

- Many apps will have meditations of different lengths; if 20 or 30 minutes seems like an eternity to you, start with something that's only 5 minutes long. On the other hand, a longer meditation may be perfect for when you're winding down at night and getting ready to go to sleep.

• Look for apps that you can listen to before buying them. For guided meditations, the most important element may be whether you like the voice of the instructor.

A SHORT BREATH MEDITATION

1. Take a deep breath, allowing your breath to sink downward, filling your belly. Exhale gently. Feel your belly and chest relax as tension flows out of your body.

2. Take another deep breath, filling your belly even more. Notice the pause at the top of the inhale, that moment of stillness before the movement of the breath resumes. Exhale. Allow any accumulated stress to gently leave your body.

3. Pause in stillness at the end of your exhale. Now inhale once again.

4. Continue for 10 slow, measured, deep breaths.

5. Allow the control over your breathing to diminish, returning your breath to its natural depth and rhythm.

6. As you allow your body to breathe normally, direct your awareness to the continued movement of your belly.

7. Focus on your breathing for 10 more breaths.

VISUALIZATIONS

Visualization is the simple act of focusing your attention on your visual sense, which can be done by looking at an object with your eyes open or looking at an imaginary object with your eyes closed. Because we are such visual beings, engaging this sense is a relatively easy way to keep ourselves focused on a single object. By focusing on a single object, we strengthen our ability to concentrate, which helps clear the mind of distractions and extraneous thoughts.

INSTRUCTIONS: EYES OPEN

1. Pick an object to focus on. In theory, it can be any object that isn't moving around too much (no animals). Common things to focus on are candles, religious figurines, or other objects you hold sacred. Objects sacred to you can be powerful, because by looking at them they inspire reverence, gratitude, admiration, and other positive feelings.

2. Sit comfortably with the object in front of you, placed in a position so your back and neck are straight and your eyes are looking directly ahead. If sitting is difficult, you can also lie down, positioning the object so it is directly in front of your gaze.

3. If practicing before bed, keep the lights dim. Sit so any light sources are not in front of you.

4. Focus your gaze on the object. Do not allow your eyes to wander. Keep the muscles around your eyes relaxed, being careful not to squint or frown. Blinking is perfectly all right.

5. Maintain this soft gaze for 5 to 10 minutes. As thoughts arise in your mind, notice them, but don't give them attention or importance. If your attention wanders from the object in front of you, simply bring it back, gently and without judgment.

INSTRUCTIONS: EYES CLOSED

1. Dim the lights, keeping any light sources above or behind you.

2. Sit comfortably, with your neck and back straight, or lie down in a comfortable position. Gently close your eyes.

3. Decide on an object to focus on, and manifest this object in your mind's field of vision (your mind's eye).

4. Continue this internal visualization for 5 to 10 minutes.

Visualization, either with eyes open or eyes closed, is a great way to re-center yourself at any time of day.

Focusing on a single object will help calm the mind and release unnecessary thoughts, and once you're finished, you should feel more calm and ready to either continue with your day or relax into sleep.

MANTRAS

Since we are very visually oriented, engaging our sense of hearing has a different quality than engaging our sense of vision. Mantras bring us further into ourselves, as sounds are often experienced as less external as compared with visual objects. Sound also generates a stronger vibration, a sensation that can permeate the body and help override and wash away any feelings of irritability, anxiety, or depression. Being able to keep your eyes closed while chanting a mantra can also help bring you more into your body, a necessary element for sleep.

Similar to a visualization, a mantra can theoretically be any sound, syllable, or phrase; however, some sounds are considered more powerful than others. These are syllables in Sanskrit, discovered to have powerful vibrations, and are known as *bija,* or seed mantras.

The syllables correspond to the chakras on the body (energy centers) and are as follows:

CHAKRA	BASIC THEMES	DISHARMONY	SACRED SOUND
1st, Root	Survival, basic needs	Fear, anxiety	LAAM
2nd, Sacral	Sensuality, physical pleasure	Restlessness, unfulfilled desires	VAAM
3rd, Solar Plexus	Personal power, self-esteem	Regret, guilt	RAAM
4th, Heart	Compassion, love	Heartbreak, sadness, bitterness	YAAM
5th, Throat	Communication, expression	Resignation, feeling stifled	GHAA
6th, Third Eye	Intuition, insight	Stuck, close-minded	KSHAAM
7th, Crown	Connection to the Divine, spirituality	Lack of awe and wonder	OMM

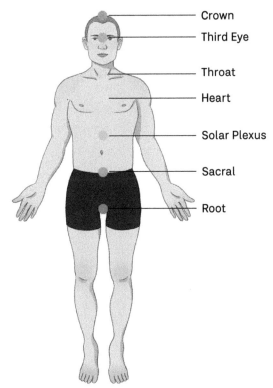

Each sacred sound resonates with its corresponding chakra, opening and increasing its energy. If you wish to use one of these sounds, I recommend finding a video or audio recording so you know how to pronounce the syllable properly. If you aren't familiar with the chakras, I would also recommend learning more about them in order to choose the best one for you to work with.

1. Choose your mantra, whether it be a sound from the list on page 64, a different phrase in Sanskrit, or just a simple English word.

2. Sit comfortably, with your back and neck straight. You can also lie down if that is more comfortable.

3. If you wish, close your eyes. You can also keep them open if that's more relaxing.

4. Begin to repeat your mantra, either out loud or silently in your head.

5. Continue for 5 to 10 minutes.

Sometimes mantras can energize you instead of helping you go to sleep. Pay attention to how you feel after chanting, and if you find a particular sound, word, or phrase makes you more alert, or more active, this mantra would be a good choice for the morning, not the evening. Experiment to find out what works for you.

BREATH AWARENESS

The breath is the one thing that must keep moving, even while we are physically at rest. (The heart also moves continuously, but most people can't feel their heart beating just by focusing on the chest.) The movement of the breath makes it a powerful tool for training the mind. We will discuss breathing exercises in the next chapter, where the breath is controlled and regulated. This section is about meditating with the breath, becoming aware of our own breathing, and observing it without judgment.

The breath is an important link between the subconscious and conscious levels of the mind. It is an aspect of the body that happens automatically, but can still be consciously controlled. The breath is also linked intimately to how we feel in the moment. When we feel stressed or anxious, the breath will speed up and become shallower. When we feel sad or depressed, it will become slow and heavy. Paying attention to the breath is also paying attention to one's state of mind.

Since the mental states that prevent sleep arise initially from the subconscious, it is important to interface with the subconscious if we want to shift these patterns. Using the breath to pay attention to these feelings helps us acknowledge these underlying patterns, and creates space for them to shift and transform. This technique is not about forcibly changing our mental state; it is about getting to know ourselves better and learning how to *accept* what we feel deep inside.

As with many meditation techniques, it is best to sit comfortably, with the back and neck straight, and eyes closed. You can also practice this technique while already lying down in bed, though it can be more difficult to focus than when sitting upright. Keep lighting dim and away from your face. If there is distracting noise in your environment, soft white noise that masks it may help you concentrate.

INSTRUCTIONS

1. Bring your attention to the natural flow of the breath, allowing your body to breathe naturally, without attempting to change the breath in any way.

2. Keeping your awareness within the body, concentrate on the movement of the breath:

   • through the nose

   • through the trachea

   • in the chest or abdomen

   • from the nose to the belly

3. Wherever you place your attention, just feel, without judging or wanting the breath to be different than it actually is.

It is common to become lost in thought during this exercise. When you notice you've become distracted, simply return your attention to the breath, without becoming frustrated or upset. Despite the simplicity of this technique, it is not easy. However, even if you only manage a few seconds of breath awareness at a time, the benefits will come. Slowly, you will gain greater and greater acceptance, which is a necessary condition for peace and calm.

This technique can be practiced anywhere, anytime, and is especially beneficial when you feel stressed, anxious, or agitated. Five to 10 minutes is a good amount of time at first; however, this technique is cumulative and provides better and better results the more you practice it. If you are especially stressed, it may take longer than 10 minutes for this technique to help you become calm. In such a case, if you have time, work with the breath for longer.

SENSATION AWARENESS

Just as the breath provides a link between the subconscious and the conscious parts of the mind, body sensation is a direct reflection of the state of our subconscious mind. Sensation here refers to whatever you can feel at the physical level, such as tingling, pressure, heaviness, itching, heat, cold, and other physical feelings too numerous to name here. Body sensation is the source of our mental and emotional feelings, which then go on to feed into our thoughts and mental impressions.

More and more, our perception and understanding of thoughts and emotions in the West are catching up with what the East has known for millennia: mind and body are so interconnected and intertwined that they are functionally inseparable. This intimate connection is why you can use awareness of physical sensation to explore and transform the mind.

Body sensation is always there, an automatic response to environmental stimuli. During our entire lives, we've used our sensations as a guide—mostly unconsciously—to decide what is good and what is bad. When something feels unpleasant, we dislike this feeling and label it as bad. When something feels pleasant, we like the feeling and label it as good. But this approach to stimuli creates issues, because we have very little control over environmental stimuli.

Lack of control over stimuli leads to lack of control over sensation; sensation, in the moment, just *is*. When you are feeling something, in that moment it is just there, and you have to live with it for that moment in time. Therefore, in a similar fashion to awareness of the breath, a critical element of this technique is to simply feel, without desiring more of a pleasant sensation or pushing away an unpleasant one. This is simple, but it can be very difficult.

When you can just *be* with a sensation, it is allowed to manifest itself without any obstructions. It takes energy to create sensations, and the body-mind does this with a purpose. By training yourself to feel sensation without judgment, the energy behind the sensation plays out with minimal interference. Thus, the thoughts and emotions accompanying the sensation are also allowed to flow, unimpeded. You learn to easily let go of agitating thoughts and emotions, such as irritation, frustration, anxiety, fear, or excitement, all of which tend to prevent sleep.

Though you can practice this technique anywhere and anytime, it is an excellent technique to use when you are already in bed. It can also be very helpful to practice this after, or in conjunction with, the progressive muscle relaxation technique described in chapter 4 (page 50).

INSTRUCTIONS

1. Begin by noticing the sensation in your feet. If you can't feel anything, pay attention to the sensation on your skin from the sheets or blankets.

2. Work your way up your body, moving from the feet to the calves, the shins, the knees, the thighs and upper legs, up to the groin. Continue to observe sensations, without wanting them to be different from how they are.

3. Keep going, moving through the pelvis, lower back, and abdomen. Work your way through your chest, mid-back, and upper back.

4. Continue to your shoulders, arms, and hands. Finish by noticing the sensations in your neck, face, and head.

If you have especially intense sensations that are obviously connected to emotional turmoil you're experiencing, stay with those sensations for a few minutes. Practice allowing them to exist without fighting against them. You will find that after a while the sensation will start to change without your needing to do anything except pay attention.

PITFALLS OF MEDITATION

Though not discussed much in popular culture, there are quite a lot of known side effects from practicing meditation, some of which can be extremely unpleasant. These side effects fall into multiple categories, including changes in mood, mental state, perception, sense of self, and relationships with others. They are more common with mindfulness-type practices, such as breath and sensation awareness, as opposed to visualization or mantra work. This is because the serious practice of mindfulness techniques is about becoming aware of, and deconstructing, the structure and foundation of who you are.

If you are a person who is anxious much of the time, mindfulness practices may reveal how anxiety has become a part of your identity. Changing this anxiety means changing who you are at a deep level, which could be very disturbing.

Though the short time durations suggested in this chapter are unlikely to trigger anything, people with a history of psycho-emotional trauma should be especially cautious and proceed slowly. You will likely find that exercises that avoid placing attention on your chest or abdomen will be okay. More active techniques, such as chanting, may be better choices than the more passive, awareness-based exercises. For breathing exercises, you may find that focusing on the breath as it passes through the nose will be okay, and give you some of the benefits without triggering a trauma response. With sensation awareness, pick a part of the body that doesn't trigger any uncomfortable feelings and avoid the chest and abdomen, which is where we often store traumatic emotions.

CONCLUSION

Though it isn't possible to fully discuss here all the different types of meditation, hopefully you've gotten an understanding of how to use the techniques outlined in this chapter, and the reasons for doing so. Meditation techniques work to help calm the mind and promote good sleep, though they can be used for much more than that. Some of these techniques may produce results for you quickly, whereas others may not suit you or may require a greater investment of time and energy to really pay off. As with the other therapies and remedies presented in this book, try a few different techniques, see what works for you, and soon you'll be sleeping better than ever. If all this mental work and focus isn't your style, the next chapter should be more to your liking, as it covers physically oriented techniques and therapies.

CHAPTER 6

BREATHING, STRETCHING, AND HYDROTHERAPY

In addition to doing the mental exercises of chapter 5, it is important to take care of the physical body in order to promote quality sleep. In this chapter, we will focus on techniques that work with the physical body, including aspects of our physiology such as the nervous system and cardiovascular system. First, we will explore the underlying principles that connect these physiological mechanisms to sleep. Just as transforming our mental processes has an effect on the physical body, working with the physical body can positively affect our mental and emotional state. Since the process of sleep involves releasing our awareness of the outside world and allowing our consciousness to descend into the body, preparing the body physically for relaxation is very helpful.

THE POWER OF YOUR BREATH

The breath has been a focus of meditative techniques for millennia. In many traditional healing systems, the breath is synonymous with life, as breathing is the one thing we must do almost continuously to stay alive. Breathing is a constant source of movement in the body, even when we are totally still or asleep. The movement of the diaphragm creates a rhythmic flow that helps circulate blood through the internal organs, especially the lungs. This is critical, since the blood of the entire body goes through the lungs with every heartbeat. If breathing is inhibited, circulation will be restricted, blood won't be as well oxygenated, and the whole body will suffer.

The breath is also representative of our ability to change and transform. Just as breathing out releases carbon dioxide, a product of our metabolism, exhaling also releases old emotions, thoughts, and beliefs. And just as breathing in allows us to absorb oxygen from the air, inhaling is symbolic of all that we need to imbibe in order to grow and evolve. As we exhale, we release what is old; as we inhale, we take in what is new. In the space between, when we are still, we reside in the present moment.

BREATHING AND THE NERVOUS SYSTEM

The breath has an intimate connection to our mental-emotional state. When we feel stressed or anxious, our breathing becomes rapid and shallow. When we feel moody or emotional, we take deep breaths and sigh, as a way to help release those feelings. When there are emotions we do not want to feel, we hold our breath. This connection is facilitated by the influence of the diaphragm over the nervous system—specifically, the link between the head-brain and the gut-brain.

It is now known that the gut contains a second brain. This body-brain, also called the enteric nervous system (ENS), is constantly communicating with the head-brain, providing feedback about the state of the internal organs. One of the major nerves that connects the brain and ENS is the vagus nerve, a major nerve of the parasympathetic nervous system (PNS), known as our *rest-and-digest* system. The vagus nerve, along with other important nerves, passes directly through the diaphragm and integrates what's happening in the ENS with both breathing and emotion. In this way, the movement of the breath has a profound influence on our emotional state.

THE BENEFITS OF FOCUSING
ON YOUR BREATH

As discussed in the previous chapter, focusing on the breath is one way to become more aware of our deeper, subconscious patterns. The first step of changing a pattern, or habit, is to become aware of it, and the breath helps us do this. It can also be helpful with actively changing patterns of emotional response. The breath can be controlled, and this conscious control of our breathing can affect some of our subconscious processes and change how we feel.

One important aspect of working with the breath is the use of diaphragmatic tension to suppress unpleasant emotions. As mentioned in the last chapter, suppressed emotion often lives physically in the chest or abdomen, and the diaphragm is a significant player in this suppression. Many people have emotions they haven't allowed themselves to feel, but there is the possibility of releasing these feelings by consciously shifting breathing patterns. If you have had traumatic experiences or carry old emotional wounds, be particularly careful and go slowly with the breathing exercises detailed in this chapter.

THE IMPORTANCE OF CIRCULATION

Though we typically cannot feel it, the heart (as well as all its blood vessels) is another organ that is in constant motion, rhythmically contracting and relaxing. This movement of our cardiovascular system distributes life-giving blood to every part of our body. Though blood and circulation are often overlooked in Western medicine with regard to sleep, in Chinese medicine the circulatory system is intimately involved in the sleep process. (See chapter 9 [page 140] for specific circulation-related insomnia patterns.)

As mentioned in chapter 2 (page 20), our core body temperature drops while we are asleep, and this is facilitated by bringing warm blood from our core to the surface of the body. This is why warming the extremities helps people fall asleep faster: it dilates the peripheral blood vessels, which draws blood to the extremities and helps facilitate the lowering of the core temperature.

Good circulation is also critical to helping the tissues in different parts of the body heal and rejuvenate during sleep. Blood brings oxygen, nutrients, growth factors, and more to the cells, and carries away carbon dioxide, old proteins, and metabolic wastes, among other things. Without this flow of blood, cells and tissues won't be able to fully regenerate. This can translate to feeling tired and unrefreshed even after a full night's sleep.

THE BENEFITS OF MOVEMENT

Movement and exercise have been shown over and over to be critical elements of good health, and this extends to healthy sleep as well. One of the main ways that movement assists sleep is by promoting good circulation. In addition to the cardiovascular system, we rely on regular movement to assist the flow of blood and other fluids in the body. Veins cannot pump blood on their own; they rely on muscle movement for good blood flow. Similarly, our lymphatic system relies on regular movement, which is why people often find that their feet and ankles swell up if they sit still for too long (such as on an airplane).

Lack of movement also leads to tight muscles, for several reasons. The "use it or lose it" principle, which applies to almost everything we do, means that without regular stretching, muscles stop being able to stretch well. Partly, this is because of circulation: muscles need fresh blood and oxygen to stay relaxed, and lack of movement hinders the flow of blood. When muscles get tight, they further compress blood vessels, compounding the issue. Therefore, proper movement and stretching is very important to promote circulation and help the body relax in the evening.

BREATHING, CIRCULATION, AND MOVEMENT FOR SLEEP

Falling and staying asleep depends heavily on being able to relax, at both the physical and mental level. Breathing exercises, optimizing circulation, and proper movement are all ways to assist this relaxation. Since the mind and body are interconnected, any of these approaches can relax our mental state as well as our physical body. You may find that one of the following techniques works especially well for you; however, every person needs to move, and every person needs to breathe. These two areas of daily life, along with their influence over circulation, can and should be optimized in every person. Doing so will go a long way toward helping you fall and stay asleep.

EXERCISES

The following exercises are designed to engage the physical body to facilitate better sleep.

DAILY MOVEMENT

The importance of regular physical movement cannot be overstated. Numerous studies have shown that exercise is important for good health and for preventing a variety of chronic diseases. Exercise is also important for good sleep at night and has been shown to improve sleep apnea and sleep quality, as well as physical and cognitive performance during the day.

The best type and duration of exercise is unique to every individual, but in general, 30 to 45 minutes of moderate aerobic exercise is a good goal. Good activities are walking, jogging, biking, or rowing; anything that engages the whole body, makes you breathe hard, and produces a very light sweat is appropriate. It's also important to try to exercise during the day, and not at night right before sleep. As mentioned in chapter 2 (page 24), try to finish any physical exercise at least three to four hours before bed.

It's important to move regularly throughout the day. Many people in today's world spend the majority of their time sitting. This is detrimental to good circulation, for the reasons we previously discussed. If you sit for most of your day, stand up at least every hour, and every 30 minutes if possible. Stretch, move around a little, and keep your body feeling relaxed and limber. Regular movement is potentially more important than exercise that is more intense but less frequent.

STRETCHING EXERCISES

Standing "Dangling" Forward Bend

This simple stretch is great for opening and lengthening the entire back of the body, from the ankles to the head. Our major fight-or-flight muscles lie along this back line, and giving them some attention with this stretch is great for relieving stress from a difficult day.

- Stand with your feet pointing forward, shoulder-width apart.

- Slowly bend forward and reach for the ground. Keep your knees slightly bent to distribute the stretch between your back and legs. Don't push yourself farther than is comfortable.

- Once you've gone as far as you can, cross your arms, grabbing the opposite elbow.

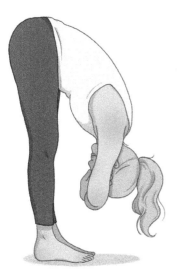

1. Allow your arms and head to become relaxed and heavy, so that their weight relaxes and lengthens your neck, back, and legs.

2. Move a little to stretch different areas. Bend one knee a little more, then the other. Gently twist your spine back and forth. Explore how your body feels.

3. When you're ready, slowly straighten back up, one vertebra at a time.

For all stretches, it is important not to push your body past its limits. Move into stretches slowly, and do not push into pain or serious discomfort. Pain is a sign that something is wrong; if a position or stretch feels painful, reduce the intensity.

Heart Melting Pose

This stretch is designed to relax and open the chest, helping the body release anxiety, stress, and tension that has built up during the day. It's also great if you habitually breathe into your chest, since it will stretch and lengthen the accessory breathing muscles in the chest, collarbone, and neck areas.

1. Find a comfortable spot where you can kneel on the floor.

2. Slowly bend forward to rest your forehead on the floor in front of you.

3. Place your hands on the floor above your head, palms down. The entire forearm can rest on the floor for support.

4. Keeping the thighs vertical, slide forward as much as is comfortable. The upper chest can rest on the ground if possible.

5. If you cannot rest comfortably on the ground, place a pillow under your chest.

6. Allow your body to relax into the stretch, accepting the influence of gravity and sinking into the floor.

7. When you are ready, slowly sit up or move into child's pose.

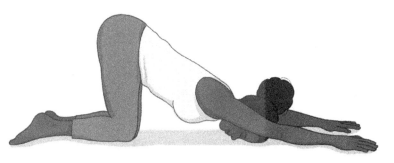

Child's Pose

Child's pose is a deeply relaxing position and can be done by almost everyone. As with all stretches, don't push yourself, and don't put yourself in any position that causes pain.

1. Sit with your legs folded under your torso, ankles and knees together, sitting down on your calves and ankles.

2. Keeping your big toes touching, widen the space between your knees.

3. Bring your forehead down to the ground in front of you, allowing your chest and abdomen to rest between your folded legs.

4. If your head does not rest comfortably on the ground, place a pillow on your thighs to support your head and torso. You can also place a pillow between your thighs and calves if sitting on your heels is difficult.

5. Bring your arms to your sides, palms up.

6. Rest in this position for several minutes.

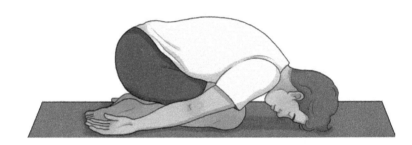

Supine Spinal Twist

Being able to rotate the body is not only important for physical movement, but also it represents the ability to see options and be flexible in our choices. Stress makes us focus on what's right in front of us, and we tend to lose sight of how things could be different. Twists are a way to help us regain flexibility, both physical and mental.

1. Lie on your back on a firm and comfortable surface.

2. Bring your legs up and place your feet flat on the ground, knees pointed upward.

3. Lift your hips slightly and shift your pelvis about an inch to the right.

4. Bring the right knee to your chest, and straighten your left leg.

5. Bring your right knee over to the left, allowing it to fall toward the floor on your left side. Your right hip should be stacked on top of your left hip. You can hook your right foot behind your left knee for support if needed.

6. If your knee does not touch the ground, simply allow it to dangle. You can also use a pillow to support the knee.

7. Straighten your arms to the side, making a T shape with your body.

8. If comfortable, turn your head to the right.

9. Relax in this position and allow gravity to pull your body toward the ground.

10. After resting for several minutes, repeat on the other side.

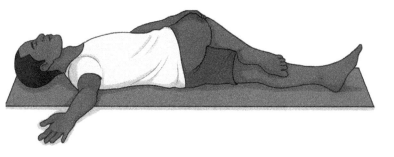

Pillow-Supported Bridge

Just as the standing forward bend stretches the back line, the bridge stretches the front line. This stretch helps open the abdomen, an area where many of us hold a lot of tension. It can also support diaphragmatic breathing by helping relax the abdominal muscles. As you'll see in the next exercise, belly breathing is an important element to relaxation and good sleep.

1. Lie down on your back and place one or two pillows directly under your hips and butt.

2. Allow your shoulders to rest on the ground.

3. You can either place your feet flat on the ground with knees bent or straighten your legs and rest your feet on your heels.

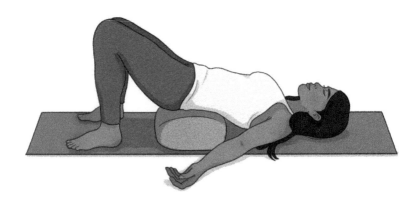

4. Allow gravity to relax your back and abdomen, giving your full weight to the pillows and the surface you are lying on.

5. Rest for several minutes or until you are ready to move on.

BREATHING EXERCISES

Belly Breathing

Chest breathing is associated with sympathetic nervous system (SNS) activation, which happens naturally when we are stressed and when we exert ourselves. This connection goes both ways: you can intentionally activate the SNS by breathing more shallowly, which triggers the fight-or-flight reflex. Belly breathing works in the opposite way, activating our PNS, which tells the body it's safe to relax. The PNS, as our rest-and-digest network, needs to take over from the SNS in order for us to go to sleep.

1. Belly breathing is best done sitting or lying down, and can be done when you are already in bed.

2. Place one hand on the abdomen over the belly button, and the other hand on the chest. If comfortable for you, close your eyes.

3. Breathe through your nose if you can, for both the inhale and the exhale.

4. Begin simply by noticing where your breath goes. If you have trouble feeling the breath in your body, pay attention to your hands and notice if they move with your breath.

5. Start breathing more into your belly, using the hand there to help guide you.

6. On each inhale, your belly should expand first and your chest should move afterward, or not at all. If your chest is moving first, or your belly is barely moving at all, keep allowing the breath to sink downward, a bit at a time.

7. Work with the breath in this way for 5 to 10 minutes.

If you habitually breathe into your chest and find it difficult to move the breath into your abdomen, don't worry. Over time, as you continue to work this way, you'll change this habit and find yourself breathing in a relaxed way more and more.

Square Breathing

Also called box breathing, this is a simple breathing exercise that can help smooth out and increase heart rate variability (HRV). HRV, as you may recall from chapter 4 (page 42), is one measure of how calm and coherent you are, and tends to go up when the PNS is dominant. When combined with belly breathing, square breathing is a powerful tool for relaxation and helps activate the PNS.

Similar to belly breathing, square breathing can be done anytime and anywhere. It may be easier to do sitting or lying down, but this is not necessary.

1. Breathe in to the count of four, hold your breath to the count of four, breathe out to the count of four, then hold to the count of four before breathing in again.

2. Breathe through your nose if possible.

3. If four is too long, count to three or even two. If you can do four easily, lengthen your count to five, six, seven, or even longer.

4. Continue this pattern for 5 to 10 minutes.

Parasympathetic Breathing

This type of breathing takes the principles of belly breathing and square breathing even further. It turns out that the PNS, and the accompanying increase in HRV, is primarily activated by long exhales. This principle is behind why we instinctively sigh when we feel emotional; the long exhale helps us release tension. You can combine the attention to belly breathing, the structure of square breathing, and the principle of longer exhales to maximize stress reduction and relaxation.

1. Begin with an inhale-to-exhale count ratio of one to two. For example, breathe in to the count of two, and out to the count of four.

2. You can lengthen your breaths as you become more relaxed. Inhale to three, exhale to six; inhale to four, exhale to eight.

3. You can also increase the ratio: inhale to two, exhale to six; inhale to three, exhale to twelve; and so on.

4. Remember to incorporate belly breathing if you can.

HYDROTHERAPY

Hydrotherapy is an excellent way to directly influence and increase circulation, and in contrast to movement and exercise, it can be done right before bed. An ancient healing technique, hydrotherapy is simply the therapeutic application of hot or cold water.

Hot Baths and Showers

Taking a hot bath or shower in the evening works to both increase circulation and help our body cool off in preparation for sleep. Superficial warmth dilates the blood vessels, and then after the bath or shower increased blood flow to the periphery helps bring warm blood up and out from our core, cooling us down and helping the body settle into sleep. It's important to allow your body to cool off after a hot bath or shower (don't go straight from a hot bath to under the blankets), but don't allow yourself to get chilled or for your feet to get cold. Taking a bath or shower can be a great thing to do before spending some time stretching or meditating.

Warming Socks

This technique is an excellent way to increase circulation throughout the night, leading to better and more restful, healing sleep. The addition of the socks creates stimulation beyond simply warming the feet, as mentioned in chapter 2 (page 21).

MATERIALS
1 pair of thin cotton socks
Cold water
Small tub, basin, or bucket
Hot water
Towel
1 pair of thicker, or wool, socks

INSTRUCTIONS

1. Wet the thin cotton socks in cold water, then wring them out until they are no longer dripping.

2. Fill the tub, basin, or bucket with hot water.

3. Warm your feet in the hot water until your feet are very warm.

4. Dry off your feet and put on the wet cotton socks.

5. Put on the dry, thicker socks over the wet socks.

6. Leave both pairs of socks on and go to bed. In the morning, the wet socks will be dry.

CONCLUSION

Given the importance of breathing, circulation, and movement, hopefully some of the exercises and remedies in this chapter will prove helpful for you. By physically relaxing the body, stimulating the PNS, and regulating your body temperature and circulation, you should be well on your way to a more relaxed state—and thus easier and better-quality sleep. The next chapter will focus on more physical interventions for healthy sleep, using the ancient Chinese understanding of anatomy in the form of acupuncture channels to calm the mind and relax the body.

CHAPTER 7

ACUPRESSURE

Acupressure is a technique based on Chinese medicine's understanding of anatomy. In ancient times, Chinese doctors, philosophers, and scientists realized that the human body is a reflection of the structure of nature and the cosmos. If we live in harmony with nature, in accordance with the environment and the seasons, and if we keep our minds tranquil and our hearts open, then we stay healthy, without disease.

However, this ideal is rarely achievable. The ancients also discovered that our bodies consist of an interwoven network of vessels and channels that have come to be known today as the acupuncture channels. The life energy of the body, known as *qi*, flows through these channels. If the qi flow is unimpeded, there is good health, but if there is an obstruction, then disease can arise. Poor sleep is one manifestation of an obstruction or imbalance in the flow of qi, and thus acupressure can help create better sleep through normalizing qi flow.

THE SCIENCE OF ACUPRESSURE

The literal translation of qi is not "*energy*"; it is "*air*." The Chinese character depicts steam rising off cooked rice, denoting the purified essence of food. There have been authors who have argued that qi should be understood as oxygen, or as electromagnetism. In Chinese medicine, there are many different types of qi, so all of these ways of understanding it are accurate. Entire books have been written attempting to understand the channels and points from a Western perspective; we will very briefly review a few concepts here.

One obvious biomedical correlation is between the channels and major blood vessels. Acupuncture/acupressure points have been shown to correspond with neurovascular bundles, that is, places where there is a greater density of tiny blood vessels and nerve clusters. Stimulating these points has been shown to alter blood flow and decrease pain by releasing endorphins.

Another structure that correlates with the channels is fascia. This stretchy connective tissue, which literally holds our body together, is organized into different planes that run throughout the body. When fascia is stimulated, signals can travel both through the nervous system and through the fascia itself, which can affect areas farther along the channel and even organs deep inside the body.

THE BENEFITS OF ACUPRESSURE

The body is constantly striving toward a state of health, doing the best it can with the resources available to it. If we are resilient, then we heal from physical injuries and recover from emotional wounds. Acupressure is about working *with* the body and helping it function at an optimum level, thus assisting the body in its natural healing abilities. Healing a cut, reducing pain and inflammation, and balancing hormones are all natural body functions; acupressure can help with these and more.

Acupressure is a great technique because most of us can perform it on ourselves. It requires very little training, and you get instant feedback from your body on whether it's working well or not. Except in the rare cases where insomnia is caused by a more serious condition, acupressure works extremely well for sleep. Acupressure helps optimize body function, and sleep is a natural function of the mind and body. It can encourage us to relax and let go of concerns, and to get much better sleep.

HOW TO USE ACUPRESSURE FOR SLEEP

Because mind and body are interconnected, physical obstructions in the channels can be both the cause and effect of things happening in the mind. As sleep is both a physical and a mental process, acupressure can be very effective for encouraging good sleep, whether by relaxing physical tension, relieving pain, balancing organ function, or helping the mind process difficult thoughts and emotions.

As you read through the following descriptions of acupressure points, there are a few things to keep in mind. If a point is tender when you press on it, it is likely more active than if you hardly feel anything at all. If you don't feel much, the qi isn't stuck, and stimulating the point probably won't change your physical or mental state. Pay attention to why you might choose to use a particular point. Everybody is different, and sleep can be disturbed for many reasons.

Acupressure Guidelines

· All of these points are best used right before bed.

· Except for points on the midline, every point exists on both sides of the body. Identify the point(s) you want to stimulate.

· Points often feel like subtle depressions or indentations. The point should feel tender, slightly "nervy," electric, sensitive, or otherwise different from a random spot on the body. If it does not, feel the area around the point (within half an inch) to see if the point is actually nearby.

- Either massage the point with a circular motion or press for a few seconds and then release. Continue for 30 seconds, making sure to stimulate both sides for non-midline points.

- Notice if you feel different in any other part of your body or if you feel different mentally or emotionally.

ACUPUNCTURE

The channels and points can be stimulated in many different ways. Acupressure is one way, and acupuncture is another, more versatile way. Acupuncture can reach structures under the skin in ways that aren't possible with acupressure, and with the use of needles, multiple points can be stimulated at the same time, something that is difficult to do with only two hands. If you want to try receiving acupuncture, keep in mind that every acupuncturist is a bit different. If your first treatment doesn't have much effect, don't give up right away. You may need to give your practitioner an opportunity to get to know you better, or you may need a practitioner who is a better fit for you.

In the instructions for finding specific points, you will see reference to a measurement called *cun*. Translated as "body-inch," it measures length relative to the size of the person. Therefore, a cun is shorter on a small person and longer on a large person. Because bodies aren't perfectly proportioned, a cun can also be slightly different depending on the body part. The following illustration provides a rough guide to this unique unit of measurement.

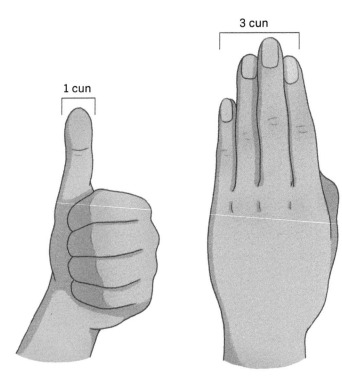

Here are a few useful anatomy terms to know:

1. Lateral: toward the side of the body
2. Medial: toward the midline of the body
3. Anterior: toward the front of the body
4. Posterior: toward the back of the body
5. Superior: toward the head
6. Inferior: toward the feet
7. Proximal: toward the torso
8. Distal: toward the fingers and toes

ACUPRESSURE POINTS

The following points are grouped by location: occipital points, forehead points, forearm points, calf points, and foot points.

OCCIPITAL POINTS

The four occipital acupressure points are all relatively close to one another. If you have trouble finding a specific point, feel along the posterior inferior border of the skull and simply massage any areas that are sensitive or tender.

Heavenly Pillar (*Tianzhu*)

The Heavenly Pillar represents our ability to hold our heads up against the force of gravity and thus supports our ability to connect to that which is greater than us (Heaven). It can become tight and obstructed when we are stressed, or when we feel like we have to keep our heads up to be aware of potential danger around us. When it comes time for sleep, however, we can't lay our heads down and rest. Heavenly Pillar can also help with tight, achy headaches in the back of the head, wrapping over the top of the head, or wrapping around the sides to the temples.

Location: Find the large depression on the midline of the neck at the base of the skull. Locate Heavenly Pillar about 1.5 cun lateral to this point, right below the lower edge of the skull, after crossing laterally over the ridge of muscle on either side of the spine.

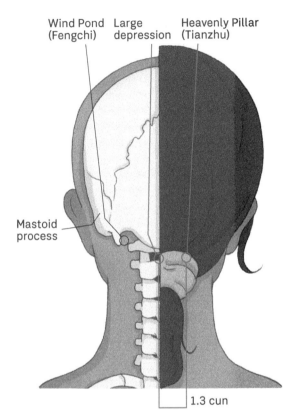

Wind Pond (Fengchi)   Large depression   Heavenly Pillar (Tianzhu)

Mastoid process

1.3 cun

Wind Pond (*Fengchi*)

A pond is a small body of water that collects but does not drain, and therefore provides a container of stillness. Here, wind represents frenzied activity and chaotic energy, especially around making decisions and getting things done. Wind Pond is a good point to use when you can't sleep due to things you have to get done or if you're feeling overwhelmed about making difficult decisions. Physically, this point helps when neck tension makes turning the head difficult, as well as for tight and throbbing headaches along the side of the head, around the temples, and behind the eyes.

Location: Place your hand on the back of your neck at the lower border of the skull, lateral to the spine. Turn your head to the same side as your hand and feel for the tendon that lifts off your neck with this movement. Locate the point in the depression just posterior to this tendon, at the edge of the bone.

Restful Sleep (*Anmian*)

Restful Sleep is considered an "extra" point, as it doesn't belong to any of the named acupuncture channels. However, its name signifies how it is used primarily to help the mind relax in order to create peaceful and restful sleep. This point is helpful for similar types of issues as Wind Pond and can be stimulated with or instead of that point.

Location: Locate the soft spot behind the earlobe, and then locate Wind Pond. Restful Sleep is located halfway between these two points, on the edge of the bone.

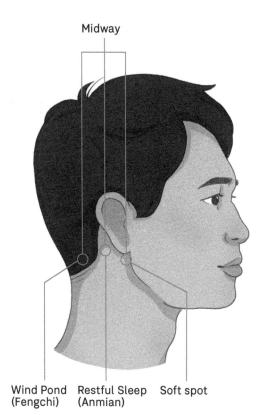

Midway

Wind Pond
(Fengchi)

Restful Sleep
(Anmian)

Soft spot

Final Bone (*Wangu*)

Final Bone can be used for similar purposes as Wind
Pond. The name, however, suggests some differences.
"Final" here can also mean complete, or finished, and
connotes the last step of something being made whole.
Bone is a symbol of solidity and structure. This point will

be helpful for making decisions and finalizing a plan of action, giving you a certainty that will help structure any actions you have to take. When it is time to sleep, Final Bone will lay to rest the uncertainty that keeps you awake.

Location: Find the tip of the mastoid process, the bony prominence just behind the ear. The point is located just posterior to this spot.

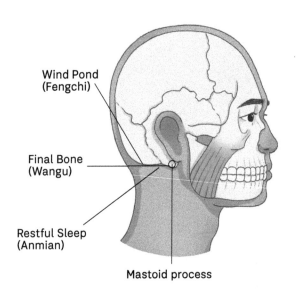

Wind Pond
(Fengchi)

Final Bone
(Wangu)

Restful Sleep
(Anmian)

Mastoid process

FOREHEAD POINTS

The two forehead points have to do with regulating consciousness and can be used to calm an overactive or chaotic mind. Don't be afraid to apply pressure, as both of these points are on the bone and can be pressed strongly.

Courtyard of Consciousness (*Shenting*)

A courtyard is where you can be outside and meet people but still be within the safety of the home. If it's time to retire to the bedroom, but your consciousness is still in the courtyard, it will be very difficult to fall asleep. This point can help relax an over-alert mind and help guide your awareness out of your head and into your body.

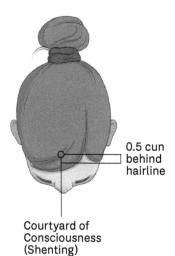

0.5 cun behind hairline

Courtyard of Consciousness (Shenting)

Location: This point is on the midline of the forehead, just above the hairline. If you have a high forehead, or your hairline begins farther back, the point may be below the hairline instead, as low as 3 cun above the spot between the eyebrows. Feel in the vicinity for a slight depression that is tender or sensitive to the touch.

Hall of Seals (*Yintang*)

A hall is the ceremonial room where the emperor places their seal on any edicts they issue. Seals were used to give importance and authority, and by stimulating this point, you can give authority to your inner intuition. The Hall of Seals is a well-known point for insomnia, and pressing it helps calm agitation and anxiety. If you can't sleep because something is bothering you, this point can help you create clarity.

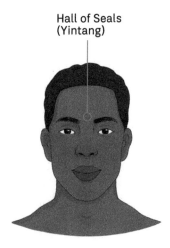

Hall of Seals
(Yintang)

Location: This point is traditionally located directly between the eyebrows. However, it can also be found about 1 cun above this spot in the center of the forehead. Feel for a subtle depression in the bone.

FOREARM POINTS

The forearm points are all close to the wrist and between various tendons. They will be easier to access if you use a small finger instead of a larger digit like your thumb. For pressure, you can use something slightly pointy, like a pen cap, if you want some extra intensity. You'll need to use enough pressure to feel the under-lying structures, but be aware that these points can be quite tender. Don't push harder than you need to.

Inner Gate (*Neiguan*)

The Inner Gate's primary influence is over the heart and dynamics of the chest. It lies on the pericardium channel, which is the heart protector, as its role is to keep stress and pain from damaging the heart. The Inner Gate is the doorway to our heart, and it can become locked shut to protect us from feeling emotions that are too intense. This often corresponds to reduced circulation in the chest and can correlate even more specifically to reduction of blood flow in the arteries and veins. This blockage in the chest can prevent sleep. You can use this point for any type of insomnia, especially if you can feel a sensation of tightness in your chest.

Location: This point is located on the inner side of the wrist, 2 cun proximal to the wrist crease, between the two tendons that run down the middle of the forearm. Some people have only one tendon; if this is the case, locate the point in the center of the forearm, immediately adjacent to the tendon.

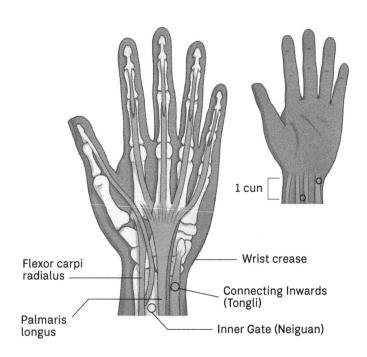

1 cun

Flexor carpi radialus

Palmaris longus

Wrist crease

Connecting Inwards (Tongli)

Inner Gate (Neiguan)

Connecting Inward (*Tongli*)

Connecting Inward is another point that is very helpful for settling the mind and connecting us back to the heart. When the *shen*, the spirit-consciousness, cannot settle inward, it becomes agitated, leading to anxiety and restlessness. Our consciousness must descend and move inward in order to rest and allow the body to focus on tasks that cannot be done while awake. You can use this point for all types of insomnia, restlessness, and difficulty winding down at night.

Location: This point is located on the fifth finger side of the inner wrist, 1 cun proximal from the wrist crease. You may be able to feel the pulse of the ulnar artery.

Channel Gutter (*Jingqu*)

Channel Gutter is an excellent point for clearing the mind. If things that happened during the day are staying with you, or if you can't fall asleep because regrets or mistakes are keeping you awake, this is a good point to use to flush those thoughts out of your head. On the physical level, this is a good point for congestion in the head, sinuses, throat, and lungs. If you have trouble lying down and feel better sitting upright, this point can help drain those congested fluids.

Location: This point is located on the thumb side of the inner wrist, 2 cun proximal to the wrist crease, directly over the radial artery. You should be able to feel the pulse of the artery at this point.

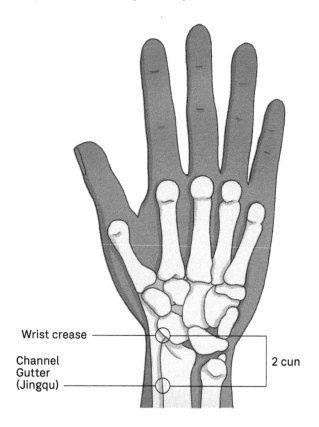

Wrist crease

Channel
Gutter
(Jingqu)

2 cun

CALF POINTS

Flexible Source (*Ququan*)

Flexible Source helps us create the substance necessary to be soft and flexible. As a major point of nourishment, Flexible Source gives us energy to be active, as well as softness to be patient. If night comes and you're finding it difficult to relax, if it's hard to stop working, and especially if you feel physically restless, this will be a good point for you. It is as if the bed within the body is hard, so it's uncomfortable to stop working and relax. This point will create softness and comfort, allowing you to relax into sleep.

Location: This point is located on the medial side of the knee, just above the crease when the knee is bent, about 1 cun toward the kneecap and 1 cun proximally, anterior to the tendons.

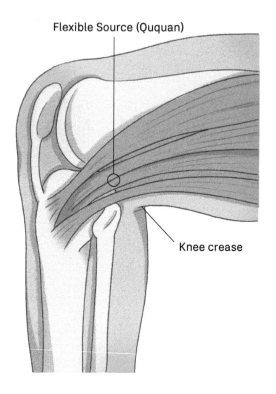

Flexible Source (Ququan)

Knee crease

Earth Pivot (*Diji*)

Earth Pivot is an excellent point when digestion becomes stuck and your system needs assistance breaking down things you've ingested. This can be food, but it can also be thoughts, emotions, and experiences. On the physical level, if you feel excessively full or it's uncomfortable to lie down because food is sitting in your stomach, this point will get the digestion moving again. On the mental-emotional level, this is a point for rumination. When your thoughts go in circles, or when you can't let something go, this point will help your mind finally "digest" and process those thoughts and emotions.

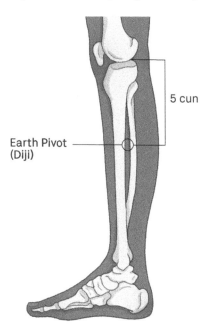

5 cun

Earth Pivot (Diji)

Location: This point is located on the medial side of the calf, at the point of the largest bulge in the muscle, 5 cun distal to the crease of the knee. The point may be close to the bone, or it may be more on the belly of the muscle. Feel for the most sensitive spot.

FOOT POINTS

Blazing Valley (*Rangu*)

The Blazing Valley point is all about containing heat and fire. In this case, the heat that the point refers to is both the heat of the body and the heat of the mind. A valley funnels and traps things, so this point can anchor heat and provide a calming influence. This point is excellent for inappropriate physical heat, such as hot flashes, and inappropriate mental heat, such as mental restlessness, anxiety, and agitation. This is an especially good point for people who sweat at night, as well as people who are both physically and mentally restless at night. If this point is right for you, it will almost certainly be quite tender.

Location: This point is located on the medial side of the foot, just inferior to the navicular tuberosity. This is the second most prominent bony protuberance after the medial malleolus and is found 2 to 3 cun inferior and distal to the malleolus. Feel for a soft and tender spot close to the bone.

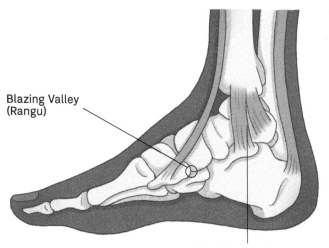

Blazing Valley
(Rangu)

Medial malleolus

Great Thoroughfare (*Taichong*)

Great Thoroughfare is a powerful point to help clear all types of obstructions in the body. The term thoroughfare refers to a canal with running water, so in addition to connection, movement, and transport, this point can also wash away stress and tension. It is very effective for all types of stress, from tight muscles to tense emotions. If you have trouble relaxing physically in the evening, or you feel like you're still carrying the stresses of the day, this point will help.

Location: The point is located on the top of the foot between the first and second metatarsals (foot bones just proximal to the toes), just proximal to the joint where the toes emerge. Feel for the most sensitive spot.

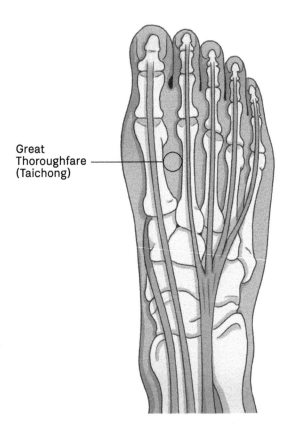

Great Thoroughfare (Taichong)

CONCLUSION

Understanding the channels and points and learning how to use them therapeutically is a lifelong process. If you can see a professional, they may be able to show you points you can stimulate at home that are more specific.

This chapter concludes the physical techniques in this book. In the next chapter, we will explore plant remedies, including essential oils and herbal teas, to help create better sleep.

HERBS AND ESSENTIAL OILS

In the previous chapters, we discussed therapies and techniques that primarily involved things you could *do* to achieve a better night's sleep, such as changing your lifestyle, moving your body, and using your mind. In this chapter, we will venture into the realm of plant medicine, which is about communicating with the mind and body at a more subconscious, physiological level. Through our oldest and most primal senses of taste and smell, plants and the medicines derived from them have played a role in human health for untold millennia.

In this chapter, we will discuss two types of plant medicine preparations: herbal teas and essential oils (EOs). Herbal teas refer to the extraction of a plant in hot water, which you then drink. EOs are aromatic, volatile (easily evaporated) compounds that are not soluble in water and are typically used for aromatherapy.

A BRIEF HISTORY OF PLANT MEDICINE

Humans have relied on plants for food and medicine over the entirety of our existence as a species. References to medicinal plants can be found in all the most ancient writings on medicine and health, and they were used in every culture all around the world. Though the original way of ingesting these plants was undoubtedly to simply eat them raw, a large variety of preparation methods have been used throughout history. Herbs are processed by drying, heating, grinding, and even fermenting them; they can then be extracted in various ways, made into powders or pills, incorporated into creams and ointments, and more. The products are then eaten, drunk, sniffed, put on the skin, placed in living spaces, and used in almost any way you can imagine.

EOs in the modern era are extracted in a few different ways. Some oil-rich plants can be cold-pressed for their oils, but most essential oils are steam-distilled. Some plants contain compounds that are destroyed by heat; these oils are extracted with a chemical solvent, such as hexane, or supercritical carbon dioxide. These EOs then undergo further processing to remove remaining solvent and any impurities.

THE BENEFITS OF HERBAL TEAS FOR SLEEP

Drinking medicinal herbal tea is the standard and most common way of taking herbs in Chinese medicine. On a practical level, making herbal tea at home requires only a pot and a stove, and can even be prepared with an electric kettle. Bulk herbs for making teas keep well, and very little preparation is needed. Herbs can be flexibly combined, and tea can be made as weak or as strong as necessary. Drinking herbal tea can help calm the nervous system, settle digestion, relax tight muscles, and quiet the mind. Taking herbal tea hot is an additional benefit, as warm drinks are more easily digested and absorbed. Finally, very light teas can also be a good source of hydration in the evening.

THE BENEFITS OF AROMATHERAPY FOR SLEEP

Our sense of smell is the sense that is most closely tied to emotion and instinct. Our olfactory nerves are routed to the brain differently from our other senses, and scent is processed more quickly, directly, and unconsciously than sights or sounds. Our sense of smell is also extremely powerful: even though we don't compare to some other animals, we can still reliably detect scents in the parts per billion range. In addition to influencing our emotions, evidence shows EOs can lower blood pressure, stress, anxiety, and depression, as well as help with sleep. By harnessing the power of scent, we can create shifts in both our physical and mental states, bringing about a state better for sleep.

STORAGE TIPS AND SAFETY

Herbs need to be protected from three main things: heat, light, and air. All of these, and especially in combination, will lead to degradation of both bulk herbs and EOs, though EOs are more vulnerable than bulk herbs. Keep your herbs sealed, preferably in darkened glass, and store them in a cool, dark place. Most EOs already come in darkened glass bottles, but if you have mixed them into a carrier oil, be sure to store this properly as well. Carrier oils are neutrally scented oils that are used to dilute essential oils so they can be used safely and effectively.

Warning: EOs are extremely potent! Unless directed by a health care professional, do not ingest EOs, and do not put undiluted EOs on your skin. Depending on the individual, EOs can cause allergic reactions if used at full strength. Always dilute an EO before putting it anywhere on your body.

There are a number of good carrier oils that can be used to dilute EOs. You will want to choose a carrier oil that is:

· Appropriate for your skin type

· Minimally refined to retain important vitamins and essential fatty acids

· Odorless or with a pleasing scent

Common and popular oils include almond, jojoba, avocado, coconut, olive, and shea butter. There are many other oils to choose from, which all have their own unique properties. EOs can also be diluted into creams, ointments, and other topical preparations. You should aim for a 2 percent dilution, which is about 12 drops of EO per fluid ounce (30 mL) of carrier oil. If you are sensitive to fragrances and chemicals, make a 1 percent dilution, or 6 drops per fluid ounce. If you want something with a more powerful scent, and you have not had an adverse reaction, you can go up to a 3 percent dilution, or 18 drops per fluid ounce.

EO DILUTION SAFETY

Some EOs are rated for less than 1 percent dilution when used topically. If you know your skin is sensitive, find an EO safety manual and look up the maximum safe concentration for a given oil before using it topically. If you sensitize your immune system by using an EO that isn't diluted enough, you may create an immune reaction that will prevent you from using that oil in the future, even if diluted to safe levels.

HOW TO USE HERBS AND ESSENTIAL OILS FOR SLEEP

For plant medicines, the most important thing to pay attention to is how they taste or smell and how they feel in or on your body. Choosing an herb or EO should ideally involve some tasting and/or smelling to see which plant agrees with you. If you don't like how an herb tastes or how an EO smells, it's probably not right for you.

Though experienced herbalists may recommend herbs for sleep be taken throughout the day, for someone new to herbs it's recommended to use them in the evening before bed. Generally, for herbal teas, it's best to wait at least an hour or two after dinner and drink the tea as part of your bedtime routine. As mentioned in chapter 3 (page 29), it's best to brew your tea with bulk herbs, though tea bags will suffice if that is what you have.

For leaves and flowers:

1. Put 5 grams of your herb in the brewing container of your choice, such as a teapot.

2. Bring 1 cup of water to a rolling boil.

3. Pour the boiling water over your herb. Cover and steep for 10 minutes.

4. Strain the tea into a cup or mug and enjoy!

For roots, barks, fruits, and seeds:

1. Put 1 cup of water in a pot. Add the herb directly to the pot.

2. Bring the water to a rolling boil.

3. Cover and gently simmer the herb for 10 to 15 minutes.

4. Strain the tea into a cup or mug and enjoy!

For certain herbs, you may find that 5 grams is too little, and for others 5 grams may be too much. If you don't have a scale at home, simply estimate, and after one or two brews you will get a sense of how much you need to use.

For EOs, there are two main methods: diffusing and direct body application. Which method you choose is primarily determined by personal preference. For diffusing, there are multiple types of diffusers, and you will need to pick one based on your preference and budget. However, avoid using heat to diffuse EOs, as this will degrade the medicinal properties. Some diffusers will require you to dilute the oil first; others will not. Follow the instructions for the diffuser you choose.

For direct body application, you can dab a drop below the nostrils, which will allow you to continuously breathe in the scent. You can also dab a drop on any of the acupressure points mentioned in the previous chapter (page 95), based on the point dynamics and the EO you've chosen. You can also use the carrier oil as a moisturizer and skin conditioner, applying it to more of the body as desired.

REMEDIES

HERBAL TEAS

All of the following herbs can be brewed as tea in the evening to help prepare you for sleep.

Chamomile
Taste: sweet, acrid, bitter
Primary action: relieves nervous sensitivity and irritability
Type of insomnia: use with difficulty falling asleep when accompanied by restless discomfort, sensitivity to all external stimuli, and unfulfilled desires

Chamomile can be very helpful to settle both the mind and the body and works well for both children and adults. Chamomile is indicated for sensitivity of the system to stimuli, where little things provoke irritability, frustration, and impatience; this can lead to whining or complaining, and a sense of wanting something but not knowing what it is. This sensitivity and irritability can lead to digestive upset or abdominal pain, as well as body pain with muscle tension or neuralgia.

Hawthorn Berry

Taste: sweet, sour, astringent

Primary action: calms nervousness and nourishes the heart

Type of insomnia: insomnia accompanied by heart palpitations, nervousness, and racing thoughts; waking in the middle of the night after sleeping well for a few hours

Hawthorn berry is an old remedy for nervousness, difficulty concentrating, memory issues, and insomnia. Like passionflower, it is both sweet and sour, but as a fruit it has more of a nourishing effect and helps when there is underlying weakness or fatigue. Mentally, hawthorn calms anxiety and restlessness, and gives the mind more energy to help with concentration. It is well known for nourishing the heart and is superlative for people who suffer palpitations or arrhythmias at night when they are going to sleep. Other key indicators for its use include dryness of the skin or mucous membranes, including the eyes.

Hops

Taste: acrid, bitter, salty

Primary action: draws excess activity in the mind and nervous system down into the gut, stimulates digestion, sedates intense emotions

Type of insomnia: use with difficulty sleeping due to brooding, intense emotions, neuralgic pain, or mental excitement (or, as a result, mental fatigue)

Hops is a powerful and complex plant, which belies its common use in beer. Hops helps sedate emotional intensity, particularly anger, and is great for intense people with red, flushed faces. It can also help calm excitement, or even mania. Hops can be useful for the fatigue, brain fog, and weakness that comes from overexcitement or intense emotion, or simply from excessive mental strain. On a physical level, hops can stimulate a lethargic digestive system as well as calm an overly hot and inflamed one. Heartburn from excessive anger, irritable bowel, and other forms of digestive inflammation can respond well to this plant. Hops is also useful for excessive sexual energy and desire, particularly in men, and can be used when this arousal prevents sleep.

Linden

Taste: sweet, moist, cool
Primary action: calms, cools, and nourishes the nervous system
Type of insomnia: use with difficulty falling and staying asleep, light sleep, or restless sleep, with inability to relax

Linden is a safe and common plant used for calming down hyperactivity, especially in children. Its cooling and moistening qualities help nourish and relax irritability in the mind and nervous system. Linden can be used for anxiety, agitation, irritability, restlessness, and insomnia when it is difficult to fall asleep or sleep is light and restless. On a physical level, linden calms and nourishes digestive complaints from nervousness, such as heartburn, vomiting, indigestion, and abdominal pain. If you have irritability (anywhere in the body) that results from feeling hot and dry, linden can help.

Milky Oats

Taste: sweet, moist

Primary action: soothes and nourishes a weakened nervous system

Type of insomnia: use with difficulty falling and staying asleep due to exhaustion and burnout

Milky oats are the unripe seeds of the oat plant and are wonderfully nourishing and soothing. They are used for all types of nervous exhaustion and debilitation, such as fatigue, difficulty concentrating, poor memory, lethargy, and weakness. These types of states come about from overwork, burnout, excessive stress, prolonged illness, and other activities that have drained the person. Milky oats will help restore your system's ability to rejuvenate.

Passionflower

Taste: sour, sweet

Primary action: gathers and soothes scattered nervous energy

Type of insomnia: use with difficulty falling asleep due to mental "noise"

This is a superlative herb for insomnia stemming from an overactive mind. It helps calm physical and mental restlessness with twitching, spasms, and general nervous sensitivity. It doesn't induce sleep so much as it relaxes and calms the mind, reducing the excessive mental chatter that prevents sleep. It can also help calm physical symptoms of nervous excitability, such as heart palpitations, hiccups, spasmodic cough, and vomiting, and help settle feelings of being overwhelmed. Physical signs to look for include a reddened tip of the tongue, cold fingers and toes, and nervous sweating.

Peppermint

Taste: pungent, cooling, stimulating
Primary action: relaxes tension, cools constrained heat
Type of insomnia: use with difficulty falling asleep due to heartburn or reflux accompanied by mental tension

Peppermint is considered a stimulating herb but can be used for situations where sleep is hindered by digestive complaints. When digestion is sluggish or there is tension in the digestive system, causing symptoms such as heartburn, cramping, abdominal pain, gas, bloating, belching, or indigestion, peppermint tea can help. Peppermint relaxes tension in the gut and helps cool the heat that tends to develop when the gut-brain is anxious. This is a good herb for times when you've eaten an overly large evening meal, or you've eaten too close to bedtime, and you experience heartburn when you lie down. If an upset stomach is accompanied by mental tension and restlessness, peppermint can help.

Skullcap

Taste: bitter

Primary action: activates digestion and internalization of stimuli

Type of insomnia: use with difficulty falling asleep due to excessive mental processing

The process of digestion is not only for material food, but is also necessary for thoughts and emotions. Our mental "food" needs to be broken down and assimilated into the body, and if this is difficult, we can feel overwhelmed by external stimulation and be unable to process it effectively. Skullcap is a wonderful herb for calming down after a stressful day, especially if you're a person who sleeps fine on slow or easy days but has trouble digesting the day's experiences if there's any stress. On a physical level, skullcap is indicated for muscle tension, spasms, abdominal pain, slow digestion, and a general feeling of constriction in the gut.

ESSENTIAL OILS

The following oils are all excellent for helping with sleep. Once understood, they can also be used during the day for the given indications.

Clary Sage
Used for: difficulty falling asleep, light or restless sleep, frequent waking, sleep disturbed by racing or obsessive thoughts, anxiety, or panic

Similar to lavender, clary sage calms the mind, but in a different way. Although lavender creates smooth movement of emotional and nervous energy by releasing tension, clary sage is more directly calming to the mind and spirit, helping calm and anchor anxiety, panic, and fear. It is also good for people who blame themselves for everything and take on too much responsibility; it helps create a stronger sense of self-worth and value in simply existing as a human being.

Geranium
Used for: restless sleep, waking after three to four hours and not being able to fall back asleep, hot flashes and night sweats, vivid or intense dreams

Geranium is a versatile and deep-acting essential oil, though it is perhaps less well-known than other oils. It is quite strong, so make sure you have a chance to smell it before using it for the first time. Similar to all the oils discussed here, it can calm nervousness and anxiety, and goes to the chest to create a sense of calm. It increases circulation and helps with overcoming sub-conscious fear that creates anxiety and agitation. It can help with restlessness at night, or difficulty falling back asleep after waking in the middle of the night.

Lavender

Used for: difficulty falling asleep due to tension and accumulated stress, or waking in the middle of the night with difficulty falling back asleep due to stress and tension

Lavender is one of the most well-known oils for soothing and calming the mind and nervous system. It works exceptionally well to relax tension in the nervous system, as well as opening the chest and unblocking the diaphragm to release stress. It also helps inspire smooth and easy movement of emotional energy, which is good for letting go of stress and tension from the day. Lavender helps quiet busyness, releasing the need for constant productivity when it's time to sleep. It can also soothe physical tension due to stress, from tight muscles to cramping and spasms.

Neroli
Used for: difficulty falling asleep with feelings of being emotionally overwhelmed; hysteria, or mania, accompanied by chest pain or heart palpitations; sleep disturbed by nightmares

Neroli is a good essential oil for more extreme emotional states that are preventing sleep. It helps clear excessive excitement and feelings of hysteria, calms nightmares and intense dreams, and relaxes the physical tension that accompanies intense emotions, such as chest pain and heart palpitations. It is a good oil for the immediate aftermath of intense or traumatic experiences, such as car accidents. When it's difficult to sleep due to feeling overly amped up, neroli can help.

Orange
Used for: sleep disturbed by anxiety, stress, hyperactivity, and nervous tension, especially if accompanied by heart palpitations or arrhythmias

Orange has become an extremely commonly used essential oil, though not always for aromatherapy, as it's often added to natural cleaning products for its degreasing properties. In the body, it can also help cut any "grease" that has built up. It is good for excess energy in the heart that leads to arrhythmias and heart palpitations, excessive excitement, hyperactivity, mania, tension, and anxiety. Orange is also relaxing to the nervous system and can clear mental confusion accompanied by stress and anxiety.

Roman Chamomile
Used for: difficulty falling and staying asleep due to feeling vulnerable and afraid

In addition to its popularity as a tea, chamomile is also available as an essential oil, though it is used for slightly different reasons. Roman chamomile is primarily for nervousness and agitation stemming from fear and a feeling of vulnerability. When you feel unsafe and vulnerable, and especially if this leads to shaking and trembling, Roman chamomile can be very helpful. It is also good for fear of being noticed by others, or fear of unwanted attention.

Rose
Used for: difficulty sleeping due to stress, tension, and anxiety, particularly due to relationship issues

Rose has long been associated with emotions and the heart, and is known for helping with stress, tension, depression, and anxiety. With its special focus on the heart, rose is also good for fear and anxiety around relationships. Of the oils listed here, it is the most appropriate for insomnia stemming from relationship difficulties, such as lying awake with thoughts centered around a relationship, or lack thereof. It is also very effective for dissipating stress and tension that has built up for any reason.

Vetiver

Used for: restless sleep and muscle spasms stemming from depleted energy reserves; waking in the middle of the night with muscle cramps; vivid or intense dreams that disturb sleep

Vetiver is another essential oil that is calming to a tense nervous system. It relaxes physical and mental tension, soothing restlessness and muscle spasms. It is particularly good when restlessness stems from lowered energy reserves that have become depleted through overwork and deep fear. Vetiver comforts this fear and provides the nourishment necessary to both relax and express these deep feelings. On the physical level, it can strengthen hypermobile tendons and ligaments, as well as relax the tension created by the body to compensate for this weakness.

CONCLUSION

The study and use of plants medicinally is a lifelong journey, and the descriptions here cannot possibly capture the full understanding of each herb or essential oil. However, with the information here, along with your own experiences of each plant, you will be able to make use of these remedies to begin sleeping easier, deeper, and better.

In the following chapter, we will examine some specific situations of disturbed sleep, with suggestions of one or more therapies that may be helpful.

CHAPTER 9

REMEDIES FOR COMMON SLEEP SCENARIOS

Now that we've explored numerous remedies for sleep issues, this chapter will provide examples of specific issues that often arise, along with techniques and remedies that could be helpful in each of these scenarios. For each situation, a few therapies from different chapters will be combined to create a realistic approach. Keep in mind that sleep hygiene practices are helpful (and sometimes necessary) for everybody in any situation. For instance, the basics of our circadian rhythm always apply, so make sure to use best practices from chapter 2 (page 14).

You're having trouble falling asleep because you're planning for tomorrow's meeting, trip, get-together, or other event.

Diagnosis: mental activity creating nervous system tension

Recommendations:

- Diffuse some lavender essential oil in your bedroom (chapter 8, page 135).

- Make a to-do list (chapter 4, page 41).

- Work with an affirmation for a few minutes, such as "I am prepared" (chapter 4, page 43).

- Do five minutes of breathing exercises (chapter 6, page 89).

- Massage the acupressure point Great Thoroughfare (chapter 7, page 117).

When you're about to fall asleep, you startle, which wakes you up.

Diagnosis: hypervigilance preventing relaxation

Recommendations:

- Drink a cup of passionflower tea (chapter 8, page 131).

- Apply Roman chamomile essential oil (chapter 8, page 137) to the acupressure point Courtyard of Consciousness (chapter 7, page 107).

- Activate heart coherence (chapter 4, page 42).

- Do some progressive muscle relaxation (chapter 4, page 50), followed by breath or sensation awareness (chapter 5, pages 66–72).

You're struggling to fall asleep because you're ruminating on things that happened that you wish had gone differently.

Diagnosis: inability to digest and assimilate experiences

Recommendations:

- Drink a cup of skullcap tea (chapter 8, page 133).

- Practice releasing regrets (chapter 4, page 44) and generating gratitude (chapter 4, page 48).

- Rumination often goes with the third chakra; chant the third chakra mantra for a few minutes (chapter 5, page 64).

- Massage the acupressure point Earth Pivot (chapter 7, page 114).

You're struggling to fall asleep because your stomach is too full, your digestion feels sluggish, or you get heartburn when you lie down.

Diagnosis: digestive stagnation and activity preventing sleep

Recommendations:

- Eat dinner earlier (chapter 2, page 17).

- Make a cup of peppermint, skullcap, or hops tea (chapter 8, page 132, 133, 129).

- Do five minutes of parasympathetic breathing to help stimulate your digestion (chapter 6, page 91).

- Massage the acupressure points Inner Gate (chapter 7, page 109) and Channel Gutter (chapter 7, page 111).

You feel a lot of physical tension at bedtime, which translates to difficulty falling asleep due to pain.

Diagnosis: tension and poor circulation creating pain

Recommendations:

- Get appropriate exercise during the day (chapter 6, page 81).

- Take a hot shower or bath (chapter 6, page 92).

- Drink a cup of linden tea (chapter 8, page 130).

- Spend a few minutes in each of the poses and stretches from chapter 6 (page 82).

- Massage some vetiver essential oil (chapter 8, page 138) into the acupressure point Flexible Source (chapter 7, page 113).

You're a light sleeper and every little noise wakes you up, but it's relatively easy to fall back asleep.

Diagnosis: nervous system fatigue hinders deep sleep

Recommendations:

· Drink a cup of milky oats tea (chapter 8, page 131).

· Activate heart coherence (chapter 4, page 42) and generate gratitude (chapter 4, page 48) to soothe your heart.

· Diffuse some clary sage essential oil (chapter 8, page 134).

· Perform the warming socks treatment (chapter 6, page 93).

· Practice breath awareness if you are awake while in bed (chapter 5, page 66).

You find yourself waking up after intense or vivid dreams.

Diagnosis: circulatory stagnation interrupting gut-brain communication

Recommendations:

· Drink a cup of hops tea (chapter 8, page 129).

· If you can identify them, work on releasing regrets (chapter 4, page 44).

- End your showers with cold water in the morning to help stimulate circulation (chapter 6, page 92).

- Practice belly breathing for five minutes before bed (chapter 6, page 89).

- Massage the acupressure points Restful Sleep (chapter 7, page 104) and Connecting Inward (chapter 7, page 111).

- Apply neroli essential oil (chapter 8, page 136) to these same acupressure points.

You feel restless and wake up every time you turn over, or you find yourself moving around a lot in bed.

Diagnosis: nervous system fatigue failing to inhibit reflexive movement

Recommendations:

- Give yourself longer to wind down at night.

- Have a small snack before bed (chapter 2, page 18).

- Diffuse some rose essential oil in your bedroom (chapter 8, page 137).

- Spend a few minutes in heart melting pose and/or child's pose (chapter 6, pages 84–85).

- Go through the progressive muscle relaxation exercise (chapter 4, page 50).

- As you lie in bed, practice sensation awareness to stay grounded in your body (chapter 5, page 69).

You find yourself waking frequently and needing to drink water.

Diagnosis: kidney/adrenal fatigue and dysfunction of circadian rhythm neurons

Recommendations:

- Drink more water during the day (chapter 2, page 16).

- Drink a cup of linden tea (chapter 8, page 130).

- Spend a few minutes in pillow-supported bridge position (chapter 6, page 88) to help your kidneys.

- Chant the mantra corresponding to the second chakra for five minutes (chapter 5, page 64).

You sleep well for several hours but then wake up, often around the same time every night.

Diagnosis: low blood sugar prompts secretion of adrenaline and cortisol

Recommendations:

· Have a small snack before bed (chapter 2, page 18).

· Drink a cup of hawthorn berry tea (chapter 8, page 128).

· Activate heart coherence to nourish the heart field
(chapter 4, page 42).

· Spend a few minutes visualizing your blood sugar
remaining stable all night long (chapter 5, page 61).

· Massage or apply geranium essential oil (chapter 8,
page 134) to the acupressure point Flexible Source
(chapter 7, page 113).

You often wake up in the middle of the night and it takes 30 minutes to several hours to fall back asleep.

Diagnosis: circulatory stagnation in the chest and brain

Recommendations:

· Get appropriate exercise during the day (chapter 6, page 81).

· Relax into Heart Melting Pose for 5 to 10 minutes (chapter 6,
page 84).

· Practice belly or square breathing (chapter 6, page 90)
while in Heart Melting Pose (chapter 6, page 84).

· Do the Warming Socks treatment to help with circulation
at night (chapter 6, page 93).

- Diffuse lavender or geranium essential oil in your bedroom (chapter 8, pages 135, 134).

You often get hot and sweaty at night.

Diagnosis: poor temperature regulation due to dysregulated gut-brain communication, reduced parasympathetic tone, or sympathetic "escape"

Recommendations:

- Reduce the temperature in your bedroom (chapter 2, page 20).

- Take a hot bath or shower before bed to help cool off (chapter 6, page 92).

- Eat dinner earlier so you sleep on an empty stomach (chapter 2, page 17).

- Massage the acupressure point Blazing Valley if you are also restless or anxious (chapter 7, page 116); the point Earth Pivot if you have digestive fullness or heartburn (chapter 7, page 114); or the point Wind Pond if you have excessive mental activity (chapter 7, page 103).

You suspect you have, or have been diagnosed with, sleep apnea.

Diagnosis: poor circulation and reduced muscle tone in the mouth and throat

Recommendations:

- Get appropriate exercise during the day (chapter 6, page 81).

- Throughout the day, keep your tongue resting on the roof of your mouth.

- Activate heart coherence before bed to open the heart and chest (chapter 4, page 42).

- Practice breathing exercises (chapter 6, page 80) and breath awareness (chapter 5, page 66) daily, making sure to breathe through your nose.

- Massage any of the forearm acupressure points, depending on which is most sensitive (chapter 7, page 109).

You're having trouble sleeping due to jet lag.

Diagnosis: perturbed circadian rhythm due to travel

Recommendations:

- Regulate your light exposure to reattune your circadian rhythm (chapter 2, page 15).

- Do not nap while it is light out (chapter 2, page 23).

- End your shower with cold water in the mornings (chapter 6, page 92).

- Make sure to get appropriate exercise during the day, preferably outside in bright light (chapter 6, page 81).

- Diffuse an appropriate essential oil in the evening, depending on how you are feeling (chapter 8, page 125).

You may not find your exact situation in these examples, and even if you do, the recommended therapies may not work well for you. Every person is a unique individual, so don't be discouraged if your first attempts at improving your sleep don't go well. Look over the various techniques in this book and try some different approaches. Ultimately, you will succeed. Better sleep is within your grasp.

RESOURCES

Online Resources
The National Sleep Foundation
SleepFoundation.org
The National Sleep Foundation is a nonprofit dedicated to advancing sleep health and well-being through education. Their website publishes numerous articles on a wide variety of sleep-related topics, and includes resources such as sleep tools, quizzes, mattress reviews, and various helpful sleep hygiene tips.

Start Sleeping
StartSleeping.org
This website is another good online resource for sleep, publishing advice, guides, sleep calculators, and other useful information, including articles on good houseplants for sleep, jet lag, sleeping with pets, and various common issues to consider.

Tuck
Tuck.com
An excellent resource for many sleep-related issues, Tuck has reviews of mattresses, pillows, bedding, and other sleep products, including earplugs, alarm clocks, APAP (auto-adjustable positive airway pressure) machines, and much more. It has sections and articles about babies and pets as well. Their Sleep Resources section is helpful and extensive.

Books

Buddha's Book of Sleep: Sleep Better in Seven Weeks with Mindfulness Meditation. 2012. United Kingdom: Hay House.
By Joseph Emet
This is a great resource if you're interested in a more in-depth exploration of meditation and mindfulness for sleep. Emet is a practiced meditator and writes in a clear and engaging voice, discussing reasons for mindfulness, common experiences, and specific action steps.

The Insomnia Solution: The Natural, Drug-Free Way to a Good Night's Sleep. 2005. New York: Hachette Book Group.
By Michael Krugman
This wonderful book by a Feldenkrais practitioner is full of exercises to help both the mind and body prepare for better sleep. It could be considered an expansion of chapters 5 and 6 in this book, and it will support any person in achieving the improved sleep they desire.

The Nocturnal Brain: Nightmares, Neuroscience, and the Secret World of Sleep. 2019. New York: St. Martin's Press.
By Guy Leschziner
A fascinating walk through the experiences of a British neurologist who focuses on sleep disorders. If the realm of more uncommon sleep issues intrigues you, this is a book well worth reading.

Sleepyhead: The Neuroscience of a Good Night's Rest. 2018. London: Profile Books.
By Henry Nicholls
This is a great book that discusses the mechanisms behind sleep and how they go wrong. Written from the perspective of someone who suffers from narcolepsy, *Sleepyhead* uses narcolepsy as an entry point into the fascinating science behind sleep and the various ways in which normal sleep can become disturbed.

The Sleep Solution: Why Your Sleep Is Broken and How to Fix It. 2017. New York: Berkley.
By W. Chris Winter, MD
A helpful book on sleep from another neurologist who specializes in treating sleep disorders, *The Sleep Solution* is heavy on the science behind sleep and is great at explaining some of the misconceptions around insomnia. However, there are not a lot of treatments detailed in the book, with the author urging the reader to talk to their doctor in many cases.

REFERENCES

Babson, Kimberly A., Casey D. Trainor, Matthew T. Feldner, and Heidemarie Blumenthal. "A Test of the Effects of Acute Sleep Deprivation on General and Specific Self-Reported Anxiety and Depressive Symptoms: An Experimental Extension." *Journal of Behavior Therapy and Experimental Psychiatry* 41, no. 3 (2010): 297–303. doi.org/10.1016/j.jbtep.2010.02.008.

Bennett Hellman, Andrew. "Why the Body Isn't Thirsty at Night." *Nature* (February 28, 2010). doi.org/10.1038/news.2010.95.

Blume, Christine, Corrado Garbazza, and Manuel Spitschan. "Effects of Light on Human Circadian Rhythms, Sleep and Mood." *Somnologie* 23 (2019): 147–56. doi.org/10.1007/s11818-019-00215-x.

Di Pilla, Steven. "U.S. Standards and Guidelines." In *Slip, Trip, and Fall Prevention,* 161–94. Boca Raton, Fla.: CRC Press, 2009. doi.org/10.1201/9781420082364.

Doherty, Rónán, Sharon Madigan, Giles Warrington, and Jason Ellis. "Sleep and Nutrition Interactions: Implications for Athletes." *Nutrients* 11, no. 4 (2019): 822. doi.org/10.3390/nu11040822.

Dunlap, Jay C., and Jennifer J. Loros. "Making Time: Conservation of Biological Clocks from Fungi to Animals." In *The Fungal Kingdom*, edited by Joseph Heitman, Barbara J. Howlett, Pedro W. Crous, Eva H. Stukenbrock, Timothy Y. James, and Neil A. R. Gow, 515–34. Washington, DC: ASM Press, 2017. doi.org/10.1128/microbiolspec.FUNK-0039-2016.

Durmer, Jeffrey S., and David F. Dinges. "Neurocognitive Consequences of Sleep Deprivation." *Seminars in Neurology* 25, no. 1 (2005): 117–29. doi.org/10.1055/s-2005-867080.

Emmons, R. A., and M. E. McCullough. *The Psychology of Gratitude.* New York: Oxford University Press, 2004.

Emmons, Robert A., and Michael E. McCullough. "Counting Blessings versus Burdens: An Experimental Investigation of Gratitude and Subjective Well-Being in Daily Life." *Journal of Personality and Social Psychology* 84, no. 2 (2003): 377–89. doi.org/10.1037//0022-3514.84.2.377.

Fenko, Anna, and Caroline Loock. "The Influence of Ambient Scent and Music on Patients' Anxiety in a Waiting Room of a Plastic Surgeon." *HERD: Health Environments Research & Design Journal* 7, no. 3 (2014): 38–59. doi.org/10.1177/193758671400700304.

Freeman, Michele, Chelsea Ayers, Carolyn Peterson, and Devan Kansagara. *Aromatherapy and Essential Oils: A Map of the Evidence.* Washington, DC: Department of Veterans Affairs (US), 2019. NCBI.NLM.NIH.gov/books/NBK551017.

Gao, Qi, Tingyan Kou, Bin Zhuang, Yangyang Ren, Xue Dong, and Qiuzhen Wang. "The Association between Vitamin D Deficiency and Sleep Disorders: A Systematic Review and Meta-Analysis." *Nutrients* 10, no. 10 (2018): 1395. doi.org/10.3390/nu10101395.

Gizowski, C., C. Zaelzer, and C. W. Bourque. "Clock-Driven Vaso-
pressin Neurotransmission Mediates Anticipatory Thirst Prior
to Sleep." *Nature* 537, no. 7622 (2016): 685–88.
doi.org/10.1038/nature19756.

Hammer, Leon, MD. *Contemporary Oriental Medicine: Concepts.*
Gainesville, FL: The Contemporary Oriental Medicine Foundation, 2017.

Hammer, Leon, MD. "Dr. Hammer's Lessons: Series One."
Gainesville, Fla.: The Contemporary Oriental Medicine Foundation, 2015.

Hammer, Leon, MD. *Dragon Rises, Red Bird Flies: Psychology &
Chinese Medicine.* Revised ed. Seattle: Eastland Press, 2010.

Irwin, Michael R. "Why Sleep Is Important for Health: A Psy-
choneuroimmunology Perspective." *Annual Review of
Psychology* 66, no. 1 (2015): 143–72. doi.org/10.1146
/annurev-psych-010213-115205.

Ji, Xiaopeng, Michael A. Grandner, and Jianghong Liu. "The
Relationship between Micronutrient Status and Sleep Patterns: A Systematic Review." *Public Health Nutrition* 20, no. 4
(2017): 687–701. doi.org/10.1017/S1368980016002603.

Keene, Alex C., and Erik R. Duboue. "The Origins and Evolution
of Sleep." *The Journal of Experimental Biology* 221, no. 11
(2018). doi.org/10.1242/jeb.159533.

Ko, Yelin, and Joo-Young Lee. "Effects of Feet Warming
Using Bed Socks on Sleep Quality and Thermoregulatory
Responses in a Cool Environment." *Journal of Physiological*

Anthropology 37, no. 13 (2018). doi.org/10.1186/s40101
-018-0172-z.

Konnikova, Maria. "What's Lost as Handwriting Fades."
New York Times. June 2, 2014. NYTimes.com/2014/06/03
/science/whats-lost-as-handwriting-fades.html?_r=0.

Lo, June C., Pearlynne L. H. Chong, Shankari Ganesan, Ruth L. F.
Leong, and Michael W. L. Chee. "Sleep Deprivation Increases
Formation of False Memory." *Journal of Sleep Research* 25,
no. 6 (2016): 673–82. doi.org/10.1111/jsr.12436.

Mariotti, Ron, and Eric Yarnell. "Melatonin and the Gut: Untold
Connection." Last modified October 13, 2006. *Naturopathic
Doctor News & Review*. NDNR.com/pain-medicine
/melatonin-and-the-gut-the-untold-connection.

Masterjohn, Chris. "Vitamin A Plays an Essential Role in Setting
the Circadian Rhythm and Allowing Good Sleep." Last
modified January 13, 2016. The Weston A. Price Foundation.
WestonAPrice.org/vitamin-plays-essential-role
-setting-circadian-rhythm-allowing-good-sleep.

McCraty, Rollin, PhD. *Science of the Heart, Exploring the Role of
the Heart in Human Performance, Volume 2*. Boulder Creek,
CA: HeartMath Institute, 2015.

Mitchell, Matthew D., Philip Gehrman, Michael Perlis, and
Craig A. Umscheid. "Comparative Effectiveness of Cognitive
Behavioral Therapy for Insomnia: A Systematic Review." *BMC
Family Practice* 13, no. 40 (May 2012). doi.org/10.1186
/1471-2296-13-40.

Onen, S. H., F. Onen, D. Bailly, and P. Parquet. "Prevention and Treatment of Sleep Disorders through Regulation of Sleeping Habits." *Presse Medicale* 23, no. 10 (1994): 485–89. EuropePMC.org/abstract/MED/8022726.

Pacheco, Danielle. "Sleep Disorders." Sleep Foundation. Updated December 1, 2020. SleepDisorders.SleepFoundation.org.

Princeton Engineering Anomalies Research (PEAR). "Engineering and Consciousness." Accessed May 1, 2020. PEARLab.ICRL.org.

PT Staff. "The Hidden Force of Fragrance." Last modified June 9, 2016. *Psychology Today.* PsychologyToday.com/us/articles/200711/the-hidden-force-fragrance.

Purves, Dale, George J. Augustine, David Fitzpatrick, Lawrence Katz, Anthony-Samuel LaMantia, James McNamara, and Stephen Mark Williams, eds. "Olfactory Perception in Humans." *In Neuroscience.* 2nd ed. Sunderland, MA: Sinauer Associates, 2001. NCBI.NLM.NIH.gov/books/NBK11032.

Raymann, Roy J. E. M., Dick F. Swaab, and Eus J. W. Van Someren. "Cutaneous Warming Promotes Sleep Onset." *American Journal of Physiology-Regulatory, Integrative and Comparative Physiology* 288, no. 6 (2005): R1589–97. doi.org/10.1152/ajpregu.00492.2004.

Rosen, Ross. *Heart Shock: Diagnosis and Treatment of Trauma with Shen-Hammer and Classical Chinese Medicine.* Philadelphia: Singing Dragon, 2018.

Rosinger, Asher Y., Anne-Marie Chang, Orfeu M. Buxton, Junjuan
Li, Shouling Wu, and Xiang Gao. "Short Sleep Duration
Is Associated with Inadequate Hydration: Cross-Cultural
Evidence from US and Chinese Adults." *Sleep* 42, no. 2
(2019). doi.org/10.1093/sleep/zsy210.

"Sleep." *Merriam-Webster Dictionary*. Accessed July 7, 2020.
Merriam-Webster.com/dictionary/sleep.

Thakkar, Mahesh M., Rishi Sharma, and Pradeep Sahota.
"Alcohol Disrupts Sleep Homeostasis." *Alcohol* 49, no. 4
(2015): 299–310. doi.org/10.1016/j.alcohol.2014.07.019.

Thornton, Simon N., and Marie Trabalon. "Chronic Dehydration Is
Associated with Obstructive Sleep Apnoea Syndrome." *Clinical
Science* 128, no. 3 (2015): 225. doi.org/10.1042/CS20140496.

Wahl, Siegfried, Moritz Engelhardt, Patrick Schaupp, Christian
Lappe, and Iliya V. Ivanov. "The Inner Clock—Blue Light Sets
the Human Rhythm." *Journal of Biophotonics* 12, no. 12
(2019): e201900102. doi.org/10.1002/jbio.201900102.

Wang, Dongming, Wenzhen Li, Xiuqing Cui, Yidi Meng, Min Zhou,
Lili Xiao, Jixuan Ma, Guilin Yi, and Weihong Chen. "Sleep
Duration and Risk of Coronary Heart Disease: A Systematic
Review and Meta-Analysis of Prospective Cohort Studies."
International Journal of Cardiology 219 (September 2019):
231–39. doi.org/10.1016/j.ijcard.2016.06.027.

Waters, Flavie, Vivian Chiu, Amanda Atkinson, and Jan Dirk Blom. "Severe Sleep Deprivation Causes Hallucinations and a Gradual Progression toward Psychosis with Increasing Time Awake." *Frontiers in Psychiatry* 9 (July 2018). doi.org/10.3389/fpsyt.2018.00303.

Winter, Christopher. "Choosing the Best Temperature for Sleep." Last modified October 9, 2013. *HuffPost*. HuffPost.com/entry /best-temperature-for-sleep_b_3705049.

Wood, Matthew. *The Earthwise Herbal: A Complete Guide to New World Medicinal Plants*. Berkeley, CA: North Atlantic Books, 2009.

INDEX

ACKNOWLEDGMENTS

My understanding of normal human function, disease, and experience would not be at its present state without the teachings of Dr. Leon Hammer, who over his long career as both a Western biomedically trained psychiatrist and a Chinese medicine doctor has illuminated and detailed the human condition, particularly at the psycho-emotional level.

I am indebted to Brandt Stickley for his wisdom and brilliance, and for being my first introduction to Dr. Hammer's lineage. I also want to acknowledge my many Chinese medicine teachers and mentors, including Heiner Fruehauf, Brenda Hood, Kenneth Glowacki, Joon Hee Lee, David Berkshire, and Gwen LoVetere.

For giving me my initial framework for understanding the integration between biomedicine and Chinese medicine, I would like to thank Dr. Paul Kalnins for his teachings and insights. I am also indebted to my many teachers of naturopathic medicine, including Dr. Gaia Mather, Dr. Pamela Jeanne, Dr. Loch Chandler, Dr. Nancy Scarlett, Dr. Tim Irving, Dr. Christie Fleetwood, Dr. Jim Sensenig, Dr. Glen Nagel, Dr. Steven Sandberg-Lewis, and numerous others.

For my training in homeopathy I wish to thank my teachers at the New England School of Homeopathy, Drs. Paul Herscu and Amy Rothenberg. They have contributed greatly to my ability to listen to people and understand what is unique in every individual. I am also grateful to my other homeopathy instructors, including Dr. Durr Elmore, Dr. Lysanji Edson, and Dr. Matthew Zorn.

For my spiritual training and insights, I wish to pay respects to S. N. Goenka, the teacher and tireless propagator of Vipassana meditation. Without his teaching of this ancient tradition, and without the retreat centers he established, I would not be the person I am today.

For their eternal gifts, including teaching me how to sleep well, I express the utmost gratitude to my parents, Yolanda Huang and Dan Peven. I would not be here without them.

And lastly, I want to thank my partner, Anna Cosper, for her unending love and support in all my endeavors. She has taught me so much: how to appreciate the small things in life, how to see the beauty in everything, and how to go to bed early.

ABOUT THE AUTHOR

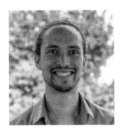 **Dr. Kye Peven, ND, DSOM,** is a naturopathic and Chinese medicine doctor currently practicing in Seattle, Washington. He received his doctorate in both naturopathic medicine and Oriental medicine at the National University of Natural Medicine in Portland, Oregon. He is the clinic operations director for the nonprofit Whole Systems Healthcare, working to create an integrative medical system focused on promoting and increasing health in addition to treating disease. He is also the clinic director for the Whole Systems Healthcare Seattle Clinic. In his practice, he focuses on restoring and optimizing the body's natural healing potential, using diet, lifestyle, acupuncture, homeopathy, and herbal medicine.